Secrets Revealed:

How Brain Science Explains Autism

And New Teaching/Parenting Methods

Secrets Revealed:

How Brain Science Explains Autism

And New Teaching/Parenting Methods

Cover design by Jerry Merritt

Dedication

I owe a special thanks to Jerry, love of my life; partner in marriage for over 49 years; Dad to our beloved son, David. Jerry is a great Dad, teaching him to use the computer, work in the yard, and cheer for Texas and Nebraska football teams. Jerry is supportive of my chosen endeavors and inspires me with his energy, drive and sense of humor. I couldn't manage without his intellectual and computer talents.

About the Author

Cheryl Merritt applies her lifetime experience in the field of autism to explain brain science and behaviors in autism with numerous real-life stories. She started the journey as a student in the 1970's at the University of N.C. at Chapel Hill with a major in behavioral psychology when the theory of ABA was at its peak. She then earned a B.S. in nursing from the University of Maryland, and discovered a fascination with patients who exhibited neurological deficits from brain injuries.

After adopting a newborn boy, David was soon diagnosed with Autistic Disorder. She taught David in the home and community. She became a trained parent leader in the family of the disabled. She has given presentation to graduate educators as well as published several articles on autism including *A.P.P.R.E.C.I.A.T.E. the Child with Autism* (copy in back of this book). She enjoys her retirement years living in North Carolina with her husband, Jerry; 33 year-old adult son, David; and three rescued cats. In 2012, she published **New Teaching Strategies for Classic Autism: Doing What Works, Doing What Matters.** She can be reached at ncbeachgirl@charter.net.

Acknowledgments

I thank my friend and neighbor, Kay Cole for taking the time to read the book, give constructive criticism and a new perspective that enabled me to make considerable changes and improve my writing. Your contribution was invaluable! I also thank my husband, Jerry, who continued to encourage me during six years of research and writing. He also provided considerable help with editing, designing the cover, formatting, and publishing. Without his hard work and guidance, this book would not have been possible.

There were numerous people who gave of themselves to help David. Terri and Domingo the gymnastics coaches whose patience, energy and persistence enabled David to experience success. David Koehn who donated his time and swimming expertise to help David experience success at Special Olympics. Theresa Moseley, the art teacher whose encouragement resulted in winning a contest for Art in the Park as well as being part of an art show with the University of Texas. Kim Nordlund Ryan, Linda Halgunseth and Claire Coats Pinkston each brought their own unique talents to share with David and they taught him about friendship. I thank the wonderful people at the Rehabilitation Hospital in Lincoln, Nebraska who welcomed David as a volunteer and gave him an opportunity to grow and learn in a work environment. I thank Polly Yarnall, our educational consultant, whose personal experience working with people with autism (especially the group homes) gave her a unique insight into how individuals can think and learn differently. When challenging situations arose, she was always there to provide support and guidance. Her work in the trenches made her a perfect consultant. Unfortunately, she died in December, 2017. She will be greatly missed.

I thank Dr. Temple Grandin, Professor of Animal Science and person with autism, for her invaluable advice over the decades given through presentations and books. I learn more from those who live with a condition than I do from any theorist or textbook. Of course, I would be completely remiss if I did not thank our son, David, who brought blessings and challenges into our lives in ways we never expected. He has taught us to view the world in a different way. His smile, enthusiasm for work and play, and weird sense of humor are greatly appreciated.

Table of Contents

Section One: History of Autism

Chapter 1
The Forgotten Past... 13
The quest to be scientific must not blind us to the past. Cheryl Merritt.
Characteristics of Victor 14; Increase Function of the Senses 15; Lessons from Dr. Jean-Marc Gaspard Itard 16; Lack of Generalization 16; Itard's Teaching Strategy 17; Dr. Edouard Seguin 18; Lessons from Dr. Seguin 19; New Label from Dr. Leo Kanner 20; Donald T. (case 1)21; Frederick Creighton (Wikky) W. (case 2) 22; Herbert B. (case 7) 22; Secrets Revealed 22

Chapter 2
The Pendulum Swings.. 25
Everybody is a genius. But if you judge a fish by its ability to climb a tree, it will live its whole life believing that it is stupid. Albert Einstein.
Creation of Mental Testing 26; Testing used to support Common Belief in U.S. 31; Testing Changes Organization of Public Schools 32; The Pendulum Swings 33; Parents of Disabled push for Social Change 34; Federal Government takes Control of Special Education 36; Attempts to Raise Intelligence 38; The Struggle to Define Mental Retardation 40; Mental Retardation in Autism 42; Secrets Revealed 43.

Chapter 3
Psychiatric Labels and Treatment........................ 47
"Most of the greatest evils that man has inflicted upon man have come through people feeling quite certain about something which, in fact, was false." Bertrand Russell.
Bettelheim and Refrigerator Mother 48; Biological Psychiatry 49; Lobotomy 49; Electroshock 51; Psychiatric Medications marketed to General Public 53; Changing and Elusive Labels 54; Psychiatry and Neurology 57; Secrets Revealed 59.

Section Two: Brain Function in Autism

Section Three: Educational Strategies for Autism

Secrets Revealed:

How Brain Science Explains Autism And New Teaching/Parenting Methods

Introduction

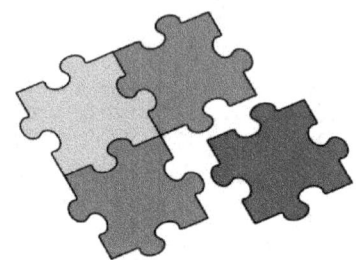

Psychiatrists have always defined autism, but it is a neurological condition. Dr. Temple Grandin and Richard Panek write in **The Autistic Brain: Helping Different Kinds of Minds Succeed (2014)**, *"Thanks to advances in neuroscience and genetics, we can begin phase three in the history of autism."* It is time to enter a new era in autism, where brain science can match the behaviors in autism with differences in brain structure and function. This book does just that. Brain science enables us to understand how the function of the brain results in children with autism thinking and learning differently, and explains why some children are higher functioning than others, thus addressing the needs of those across the spectrum.

In 2013, the label of "autism spectrum disorder" was created by psychiatrists and is defined in the Diagnostic and Statistical Manual of Mental Disorders (DSM) published by the American Psychiatric Association. The psychiatric definition of autism describes deficits with language and social interaction and repetitive behaviors, but this does not describe the needs of those with autism.

Typical children learn through observation and imitation and it is difficult to understand a child with autism who learns differently. Brain science connects the lack of observation and imitation (sensory processing

1

difficulties) in those with autism with a lack of long-distance wiring in the brain. Many symptoms, such as difficulties with memory and learning, lack of generalization, lack of exploratory play and pretend play, can be explained by the structural and functional differences in the brain. Brain science demonstrates the severity of autism correlates with the severity of abnormalities in brain structure and function, so we can now begin to address the needs of those across the spectrum.

Science reveals how sensory processing difficulties are a core feature of autism and many behaviors are indicative of this difficulty. Sensory processing difficulties can result in "blind but can see" and "deaf but can hear." As a nurse, I can mix science with intriguing real-life examples of neurology patients who demonstrate behaviors resulting from specific brain differences. I homeschooled my child, so I have many examples of behaviors that relate to brain differences. You don't have to study the brain in order to understand how your child thinks and learns differently, because you will learn through easy to understand stories and examples.

Educators have been trained in normal development of children and they assume all children follow a normal developmental pattern and learn the same way. Most educators have been taught that babies are born as blank slates and we teach them everything they know. Educators and parents intuitively teach by observation and imitation, because most of us learn that way. If the child does not respond in the expected manner, an educator assumes that the child is not paying attention or not motivated. Temple Grandin and Richard Panck write in **The Autistic Brain: Helping Different Kinds of Minds Succeed** (2014) *"Putting kids who are on the spectrum in the same classroom as their nonautistic peers and treating them the same way is a mistake."*

Changing an entrenched belief system is slow and difficult. Science often reveals truths that are less than self-evident and difficult to accept. In the early 17th Century, Galileo claimed that the earth spun on its axis and orbited the sun. He was asking people to believe something that defied common sense because it looks like the sun is going around the earth, and you can't feel the earth spinning. Galileo was put on trial and forced to recant.

Brain science now teaches that babies are born with brain cells that enable them to observe and imitate within the first hour of birth – if the brain is wired properly. Brain deficits are hidden and unless you know how the brain processes information and how a child with autism learns differently, then it seems like common sense to teach the child to observe and imitate. Just as Galileo discovered, changing an entrenched belief system is difficult.

Professionals tend to play in their own sandbox and fail to consider evidence outside of their specific area. The National Research Council writes in **Teaching Children with Autism** (2001), *"Knowledgeable researchers in one area of autistic spectrum disorder may have minimal information from other perspectives, even about studies with direct bearing on their findings."* Therefore, it is not surprising that educators and researchers fail to examine autism from a variety of perspectives. We cannot explain the puzzle of autism when professionals only examine one piece of the puzzle and they cannot agree on the condition. Therefore, to reveal the secrets of autism, we must examine various perspectives to find the puzzle pieces that fit together.

You may be familiar with the story of the blind men examining the elephant. Each person examined a specific area of the elephant. One concluded it was a fan (ears); another concluded it was a tree (leg); another said a snake (trunk); and, another claimed it was a rope (tail). They could not agree, because each man developed his own version from that limited experience and perspective.

The book is divided into three sections: History, Brain Function and Teaching Strategies. The first section examines history of autism from the perspectives of psychiatry, psychology, education, research and sociopolitical changes. It is revealing to see how our attitudes and treatment of the disabled changes over time. This enables one to throw away pieces of the puzzle that do not make sense and focus on the pieces that create greater understanding.

Section One – History of Autism

Before we can reveal the secrets of brain science to describe autism, we need to review the history of autism. If we don't know history, we may repeat the mistakes of the past. In addition, it is important to review how our society has identified and treated people with disabilities. This enables us to understand why some professionals continue to treat children in an outdated manner, based on old perspectives.

My research has revealed many secrets of the disorder that have been ignored or forgotten. Most histories start with Dr. Leo Kanner in 1943, but medical doctors in the late 1700's and early 1800's were the first professionals to educate children with autism and publish their results.

Chapter 1, **The Forgotten Past**, discusses what these early professionals knew about autism and how to treat it, based on their publications. They identified the lack of observation and imitation and lack of generalization (transferring information from one situation to another) and they discussed how they created teaching strategies to support these children's needs. They identified the abnormalities with sensations – sensing the environment through sound, sight, touch, taste and smell. These doctors focused treatment on the sensory processing difficulties, using the strongest sense to teach. This information is an important piece of the puzzle, since sensory difficulties are not considered a core feature of autism and have been ignored.

Chapter 2, **The Pendulum Swings**, explores the changing sociopolitical attitudes toward people with disabilities. History shows how changing perspectives toward people with disabilities changed our treatments for them. These attitudes influence how professionals theorize the causes of disabilities and if and how they treat them. Knowledge of history is important to understand how we arrived at today's treatment of children with autism and the mistakes we have made along the way.

Chapter 3, **Psychiatric Labels and Treatment**, reveals how psychiatrists developed and changed the label of autism many times during the 20th and 21st centuries. They do not include neurology (brain science) in the diagnostic description, despite the fact it is a neurological impairment and brain science has made great progress since the 1990's. My research reveals that there was a rift between neurology and psychiatry in the late 1800's that seems to have continued into the 21st century. When Asperger's Syndrome was added to the DSM, and the diagnostic criteria for Autistic Disorder, was expanded to include more children, this resulted in increased available monies for research and services. When Asperger's Syndrome was combined with all the pervasive developmental disabilities, the "Aspies" did not like being associated with the lower functioning on the spectrum. "Aspies" are touted as quirky geniuses and the media loves this perspective. The DSM IV and DSM-5 diagnostic criteria for autism, is printed in the back of the book.

*Chapter 4, **Applied Behavior Analysis (ABA),*** discusses the 1987 Ivar Lovaas UCLA study that is often cited as the science behind the intervention. Dr. Lovaas claimed 9 of the 19 children in his experimental group were "recovered" based on increased intelligence scores and attendance in a regular classroom. Dr. Lovaas intended his ABA program to be taught to parents, but professionals steered it to an industry specialty where only specialists could provide the service at great expense to parents. A vast industry has appeared providing behavior therapy as beneficial for children with autism, despite the lack of studies to compare it to other approaches. This industry reflects how professionals often ignore science outside of their specialty.

Chapter 5, ***Educational Research***, discusses how government research funds made available starting in the 1960's created university affiliated laboratory schools that enabled researchers to develop teaching approaches for children with autism. This created a group of professionals competing for grants with a vested interest in demonstrating success with their teaching strategies. Despite the lack of comparative studies, all the current teaching strategies are considered "scientific best practices." Most of the strategies are based on ABA (applied behavior analysis). The researchers only use high functioning students, because they are easier to work with and can demonstrate better progress, but it ignores the rest of the spectrum of autism. In addition, I show how these strategies are developed in ideal conditions and do not extend to public schools, because it is very expensive to have a specialist come to train public school educators.

Section Two – Brain Function and Autism

The second section of the book examines brain function from different perspectives – sensations and perceptions, structure and function, and memory and learning. Although most scientists do not study science outside of their specific area, I have looked at brain research from a variety of approaches – genetic, individual cells, post-mortem brain examinations, chemicals transmitting messages from brain cell to brain cell, brain imaging and studies from patients who have experienced brain impairments, such as split-brain, tumors, strokes, and trauma. Surprisingly, the various areas of research all support the same core symptoms of autism. Brain science confirms the symptoms of lack of observation and imitation, lack of pretend play and exploratory play, and lack of generalization based on abnormal brain structure and function.

You will not need to learn extensive anatomy and physiology to understand the basic differences in brain function. I will use numerous examples of patients who exhibit symptoms associated with specific brain impairments to create a clear picture of how brain structure and function affects thinking and learning.

Our learning abilities depend on the structure and function of the brain and that depends mainly on our genes. During pregnancy, genes direct the movements of cells that build the structure and function of the brain. Autism is the result of multiple genetic problems and all these genes have not yet been identified. Most of these mutations are harmless, but sometimes, they cause significant problems. Not every person will have the exact same gene mutations, so not every person will have the exact same symptoms or the same severity of symptoms.

Many professionals have made claims that they can cure children with autism. There is no cure for autism at this time, but the type of education can make a significant difference in the child's ability to be more independent and self-sufficient as an adult.

Brain research can now explain why some children with autism are higher functioning than others. For example, research shows that brains of people with autism are over-connected locally and lack long-distance connections throughout the brain to enable them to process information.

Dr. Temple Grandin, a professor at Colorado State and a person with autism, has allowed researchers to perform various tests on her brain. She has more long-distance connections and this enables her to function more independently and with greater communication than individuals with classic autism. She has also found a way to use her strength of visual imagery to compensate for deficits in memory and meaning.

We can learn much from Temple Grandin as she has shared her experiences through books and lectures. It is unfortunate that sometimes professionals view individuals with autism as subjects and not informants. I have read all her books and will show how her information is confirmed by brain science.

Chapter 6. **Sensations and Perceptions**, discusses the difference between sensations and perceptions and how we can all have different responses to various sensations. Over 200 years ago, Drs. Itard and Seguin identified how difficulties with sensations affected the child's ability to learn and how we need to teach to the sensory strength and support the weaknesses. Dr. Temple Grandin has been telling us for decades that the problems with sensory processing are significant and should be studied, but this aspect of autism has been largely ignored.

Perception is the interpretation of these incoming sensations and it relies on brain function. When a brain has altered structure and function then perceptions will be different. It is difficult for most of us to comprehend how someone with different brain function perceives the environment, but with numerous examples of symptoms from patients with specific brain differences, this becomes easier to imagine.

Chapter 7, **Brain Function and Autism**, discusses how neurological research – beginning with the decade of the brain in the 1990's – reveals the brain strengths and weaknesses in children with autism. Structure and function cannot be separated. Changes in structure will change the function of the brain and this alters the behaviors of the individual. Brain studies indicate the structural differences in autism. Comparing individuals with neurological brain deficits to the normal brain enables us to identify the function of various structures in the brain.

Chapter 8, ***Memory and Learning,*** explains how learning relies on memory. People with autism have difficulties learning and storing new information into memory. I will discuss two types of learning: associational and rote. People with autism have strong rote memories and this is based on doing something over and over until it becomes automatic, so you don't have to think about it. Associational learning relies on long-distance connections in the brain to combine details with main ideas or concepts.

There are patients who have had the long distance connections severed by surgery to prevent epileptic seizures, and researchers found this resulted in the brain processing details (right brain) but without the proper connections, the brain is unable to process main concepts from the details. I present numerous examples to connect the symptoms of autism with brain differences in memory and learning.

Section Three –Educational Strategies for Autism

There are four chapters in this section that explain what to teach, how to teach and why you are teaching it based on brain science. It also explains how teaching is individualized based on the sensory strengths and weaknesses of the individual.

In Chapter 9, ***Learn Differently; Teach Differently***, I will connect the brain functions in autism with new teaching strategies that support the brain differences and teach to the strengths. You will learn how to teach with the use of visuals, music and touch. Children with autism do not learn through symbolism (language) so we teach them "to do" rather than "to know." Many examples of behaviors you may encounter while teaching are included, and the connection to the brain structure and function is explained. A thorough discussion of teaching the child to communicate is included based on individual learning needs.

Children with autism have strengths with attention to detail and rote memory. Therefore, tasks need to be broken down into details (steps) and taught to rote memory. In the last three chapters, I include teaching charts that break tasks into steps and show how to individualize the teaching to the child. The charts are designed for the more severely challenged and can be easily adapted for higher functioning children. The strategies are not mere theory, but demonstrate real-life challenges that can occur during teaching, along with explanations for understanding and meeting these challenges. The charts enable different people to teach the child and keep updated with the necessary supports. I also explain how easy it is to evaluate progress and adjust teaching.

I created the mnemonic called **C.H.O.R.E.S.** for teaching tasks to children with autism. I use this method to demonstrate how to teach self-help skills, chores, and routines in community environments.

The mnemonic stands for:

<u>C.</u> *Charts* are used to break the task into details.

<u>H.</u> *Have Success in the Plan* by simplifying the task for the child to understand, using the child's interests, and teaching real-life skills.

<u>O.</u> *Organize Materials and Simplify Instruction* that support the child's learning needs to understand what is expected. Materials need to be organized and visual to support the child's memory deficits.

<u>R.</u> *Rely on Child's Learning Strengths* to relate meaning to the task in a manner the child can understand. Learning strengths can include visuals, music, touch, attention to details, and rote memory.

<u>E.</u> *Every Skill needs to Generalize* discusses how to help the child generalize the task from one environment to another.

<u>S.</u> *Strive for Independence* discusses how to teach so the child does not rely on someone talking him through the task, or doing something for the child. Progress on each task is evaluated based on the long-term goal of independent functioning as an adult.

In *Chapter* 10, **Teaching Self Care and Chores ,** I discuss how to create structured teaching situations, as well as how to teach handwashing, dressing, and preparing meals. Schedule examples are included to show you how to link self-care skills together into a routine that facilitates independence by teaching to rote memory.

Chapter 11, ***Teaching Life Skills in Community Environments,*** provides charts and real-life examples of teaching chores, grocery shopping, and routines for cafeterias, sit-down, fast-food restaurants. Chores include laundry, bed making, setting the table and vacuuming. Teaching in community environments is important to compensate for the lack of generalization: the ability to transfer skills from one setting to another. The long-term goal is to become more independent and self-reliant as adults, so children with autism need to be taught skills in a variety of places.

Chapter 12, **Teaching Recreation and Job Skills**, discusses the need to teach the child the skills needed as an adult. The skills are first taught one-to-one and then transferred to a group, where the focus becomes teaching social behaviors. Structured tasks are taught to enable the child with autism to function in social environments, without requiring extensive social communication or interaction.

As a parent of an adult child with an autism spectrum disorder (classic Kanner autistic disorder), I have experienced the desperate search for understanding my child and helping him succeed. Parents of newly diagnosed children all struggle with the myriad cures of the month, fearing if we leave a stone unturned, we will fail our child. In our search to understand our child, we are told *"they are all different."* In addition, families are often told that treatment needs to be provided by a specialist, at great cost to the family. I hope this book makes the journey easier for the next generation of parents facing the joys and challenges of a child with autism.

It is my earnest hope that the reader will find **Secrets Revealed: How Brain Science Explains Autism and New Teaching/Parenting Methods**, an easy read that explains the condition of autism from various perspectives, including how brain science enables us to understand how the function of the brain results in children with autism thinking and learning differently.

The extensive examples of practical, immediately effective teaching strategies, based on brain science, are not complex and are not infused with psychobabble, so they should help parents and educators quickly and easily support the child to learn important life skills. The teaching routines enable parents and educators to evaluate progress easily and reliably. This information is vital for anyone working with children with autism, including parents and educators. As Albert Einstein said, *"Everybody is a genius. But if you judge a fish by its ability to climb a tree, it will live its whole life believing that it is stupid."* I can be contacted at ncbeachgirl@charter.net. Please feel free to share the information in the book, with a citation of its source.

Cheryl S. Merritt, 2018

Note: I use the pronoun "he" when referring to a child with autism, although females can also have autism. For clarity, I use the pronoun "she" when referring to a typically developing child.

Rather than refer to the label as "autism spectrum disorder," I will continue to refer to the condition simply as "autism."

Section One: History of Autism

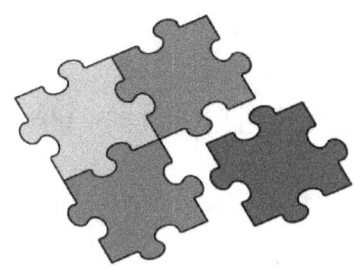

Chapter 1

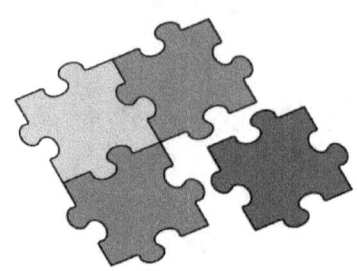

The Forgotten Past

The quest to be scientific must not blind us to the past. Cheryl Merritt

Autism is not a new phenomenon. Although most histories of autism begin in 1943 when Dr. Leo Kanner was credited with the identification of a childhood condition he labelled *"early infantile autism,"* this condition did not suddenly appear in the twentieth century. He called it *"autism"* from *"autos,"* meaning *"self,"* as he was impressed with the *"self-aloneness"* of these children.

While doing research for this book, I was surprised to learn that this disorder had been clearly described in the very beginning of the 1800's by Dr. Jean-Marc Gaspard Itard (1775-1838), who worked intensely to educate a young man named Victor with a condition called *"idiocy"*. The term *"idiot"* comes from Greek meaning *"private person"*. *"Self-aloneness"* and *"private person"* both describe the same condition.

It was physicians who initially educated children with disabilities and Dr. Itard was an experienced educator, who was the director of the National Institution for Deaf-Mutes in Paris. He devised several new methods for educating and treating the deaf, by communicating through vision and touch. Environmentalists, also known as empiricists, believed this demonstrated that intelligence is learned, and mental retardation can be cured by teaching- despite the fact that the children were deaf-mute, and not retarded.

When a young boy – about 12 years old - was found living in the woods outside Paris, responsibility for the child's welfare fell to the Institute for the Deaf and Dumb and he was confined to the care of Dr. Itard. When he was brought to Paris, he became an object of fascination. People thronged to see the *"savage"*. What they saw was a dirty, young, scared, nonverbal child who rocked back and forth.

Although rejected by other physicians as *"an incurable idiot,"* Itard felt that he could educate him and make him a "normal" human being, so he took him in and worked with him for five years, documenting his work with the boy in **The Wild Boy of Aveyron**, published in two parts, in 1802 and 1806. He named the boy *"Victor."*

Characteristics of Victor

The following are some characteristics of Victor that were revealed by Itard and should be familiar to anyone who has some knowledge of autism. Although these are all characteristics of people with autism, the current medical diagnosis focuses on communication, socialization and behavior. For decades, Dr. Temple Grandin stressed the difficulties with sensory issues and these were clearly identified by Dr. Itard. Sometimes, we think we are so advanced that we can ignore history. Forgetting the lessons of the past has resulted in education for children with autism going wrong.

1. **Need for Order or Sameness**. Itard noted Victor would return items that had been moved to their proper place.

2. **Using someone's hand as an instrument**. Victor would take someone by the hand or arm and lead them to his desired object.

3. **Not using toys in the usual manner**. Itard tried for hours to get Victor interested in toys that would be commonly used by children of his age, but with no success.

4. **Lack of gestures**. Itard noted that Victor lacked facial expression and use of body gestures.

5. **Lack of eye contact**. Itard described Victor's lack of eye contact as "expressionless" and failing to focus on people.

6. **Strange movements**. In describing Victor, Itard wrote that he would display bursts of laughter and repetitive swaying. He also had a joyful leap.

7. <u>Lack of observation and imitation</u>. Keeping in mind that Itard's experience was with teaching deaf mutes, he reported on a comparison of Victor's learning to the learning of deaf mutes. He states Victor was more challenging to teach because of his lack of observation and imitation. Brain science has now demonstrated that we all learn by observation and imitation starting as newborns. Education today has failed to recognize that people with autism do not learn in this manner.

8. <u>Lack of generalization</u>. Generalization is when a child learns a skill and then he is able to perform the skill in a variety of environments. Without generalization, the list of skills learned will have no real-life significance for the child. Itard struggled with this challenge and I will discuss it further later in the chapter.

9. <u>Disturbed by voices</u>. Victor was described as disturbed by voices outside of his room and he would check the door to make sure it was closed and latched. Temple Grandin wrote in ***The Autistic Brain (2014)***, that she was disturbed by voices outside of her apartment. She said she would listen to New Age music to block the sound.

10. <u>Abnormalities of Sensations</u>. Victor was noted to not respond to hot and cold; had limited taste preferences; preferred to smell things; did not respond to loud noises, but would respond to the cracking of a nut, which was a familiar sound to him.

Increase Function of the Senses

Dr. Itard created exercises to increase the function of each sense – hearing, sight, touch, and taste. Since Victor was known to smell everything, Dr. Itard apparently felt no need to develop this sense. He reported meager success with the sense of hearing, but greater success with Victor perceiving written words and even writing.

Dr. Itard was surprised at the benefit of training the sense of touch. First, he was able to help Victor distinguish hot and cold, roughness and smoothness. When Victor was unable to identify chestnuts and acorns by their shape, Itard noted that this sense was still untrained. Itard stated he had Victor practice comparing objects through the sense of touch, such as a stone and a chestnut. Although it was slow and difficult teaching Victor through the sense of touch, it did seem to improve Victor's attention.

Victor did not like sweets like most children, so Itard decided on a different approach to improve his sense of taste. He took Victor out to eat where all his favorite dishes were available on the table. He also had Victor sample and differentiate an acid liquid (pickle juice) from a sweet liquid. When Itard began teaching Victor to perceive different tastes, he noted this enabled Victor to eat other foods that he had always avoided.

Itard reported an improvement in all the senses with the exception of hearing. He felt that instruction of the senses had proved beneficial to Victor's education, because Victor could attend to everyday objects through the use of touch, as well as distinguish them. In addition, the sense of taste was developed, so Victor could appreciate a wider variety of foods.

Lessons from Dr. Jean-Marc Gaspard Itard

Itard struggled with Victor's inability to generalize learning from one setting to another until he discovered the need to teach practical skills Victor could use to function in a variety of environments. Itard also had to compensate for Victor's lack of observation and imitation by teaching visually (with objects and written words) and through touch.

Lack of Generalization

Generalization occurs when a skill learned in one environment extends to other environments. Typical people generalize easily, but people with autism do not observe and imitate, so they do not learn naturally in a variety of environments. Today, we have children leaving the school system that cannot generalize skills learned in a classroom to the real world, because educators have forgotten the lessons from the past. Itard struggled with lack of generalization and he provides a good description of this problem that educators face, when teaching children with autism.

Itard taught Victor to identify various objects located in Victor's room by matching with the printed word. One day, he tried to get Victor to identify the same objects in a different location (Itard's office), but Victor was unable to identify the items. In other words, Victor had failed to generalize the identification of objects to another location. Itard noted that when he placed the items on a table in front of him, Victor was still unable to identify them.

Itard then returned to his original approach. He created a single label for each object. When he put a label into Victor's hands, he still could not identify the objects with the labels. Itard attributed the failure of generalization to his training program and tried another approach. When he taught Victor to use practical objects in real-life situations, it created a meaningful experience for him. Itard was teaching him "to do" rather than "to know." He was connecting meaning with the use of an object, not just a label to an object.

The lack of generalization occurs because the child is unable to observe and imitate, and attach meaning to what he sees. Itard said working with deaf mutes was much easier and this is understandable, because they could attach meaning to what they were seeing, but Victor could not: he needed to be taught meaning with objects.

Itard's Teaching Strategy

Since Victor was unable to attach meaning to what is observed, Itard discovered a different teaching strategy to work with him. He would take Victor's hand and put the student through the motions, along with using written words and not talking. Let's look at how he does this to teach the concept of "big" and "little."

In order to ensure that Victor was focusing on the concept, Itard would take his hand, and place it where he wanted him to look. Itard selected two books that looked alike except for size. He wanted to teach Victor the concepts of "big" and "little." With the small book, he took Victor's hand and put it flat on the cover, which it hid almost entirely. Then with the large book, he took Victor's hand and placed it on the cover, so his hand only covered half of it. Itard showed him the part that remained uncovered and tried to get him to stretch his fingers to cover it, which he could not do.

Itard placed cards with the name "book" on the two books. On two other cards, he wrote "big" and "little" and placed them on the respective books. He removed the cards, mixed them up and gave them to Victor to place on the books, which he did correctly.

Itard knew that he could never be certain Victor had learned what he intended to teach, so he had to apply the same concept to numerous items. He also used the same technique to teach other concepts, such as color and weight.

We tend to teach children through spoken language, but many children with autism need to learn the meaning of concepts through touch and the written word. The child needs to be an active participant in the learning and the concept being taught needs to be meaningful to the child. Itard's experience teaching deaf children proved helpful when teaching Victor, because he relied on visual cues and not language.

Itard learned that everything had to be taught and everything had to be specific. He realized Victor had difficulties associating more than one label to an object – such as big and little for books, as well as applying one label to multiple objects.

Itard broke a book apart, so he could show Victor the separate parts – the cover and pages. As he gave Victor the part, he wrote the name on the blackboard. After some practice, Itard put the book back together and asked Victor for the names of the parts, while he touched the part. Then he asked him for the name of the whole - without touching any of the parts - and Victor pointed to the word "book". Itard wrote that he was careful to avoid confusion by touching the parts when asking the names of the parts, and when asking for the whole, he made a vague gesture toward it without touching it.

After five years of working with Victor, what was the outcome? Victor developed a considerable reading vocabulary. He lived like a human being – clean, and able to understand much that was said to him. He was attached to his caretaker, Madam Guérin. It was noted that he performed several domestic chores, including chopping wood and setting the table at dinner. Itard reported Victor could express his wants and understand directions given him. Victor continued to enjoy the open country and lacked interest in social life. Victor was quite attached to Madam Guérin and continued to live with her until his death in 1828, at about forty years of age. Itard died ten years later in 1838.

Dr. Edouard Seguin

Edouard Seguin (1812-1880) studied with Itard (this was after his work with Victor), in France, and moved to the United States to work with Dr. Samuel Gridley Howe, Dr. Hervey Wilber and others in developing training schools. He developed his "Physiological Method" of treating idiots (label for autism) and promoted it with great enthusiasm. He writes in his 1866 publication, ***Idiocy and Its Treatment by the Physiological Method***, that idiots could be cured by his physiological method.

Dr. Seguin identified the characteristics of idiocy (autism) as sensory abnormalities, such as reduced response to hot and cold; limited imitation of the body; speech but not language; sees by chance but never looks; appetite limited to a few things; disordered movement and gesture; attachment to strange objects; distant gaze; and didn't seem to cry. These descriptions are appropriate for children with autism today.

In 1876, six physicians who represented the various training schools for idiots formed the *"Association of Medical Officers of American Institutions for Idiotic and Feebleminded Persons."* Their mission was the treatment of "mental deficiency" to return the children to fully participate in their social and work communities. Dr. Seguin was the organization's first president. Seguin noted that his students - these idiots – could leave their *"will to loneliness"* and achieve independence and association with others.

Lessons from Dr. Seguin

1. **Learning should be Fun and not Stressful.** Seguin demonstrated his care and concern for the children in his teaching philosophy when he wrote that we must provide music and pleasure to children, as *"children will not be sick if they laugh"*. Seguin wrote that new things should be presented slowly and memory exercises do not help the children. If we cause stress to the child, then we should remember we are at fault, and take the child to enjoy music or pleasant exercises. Sometimes in our desire to cure, we push children to perform to a teacher many hours per day, forgetting that our actions may be causing some of the unwanted behaviors. We must not forget to have fun and enjoy our children.

2. **Teach Speech with Music**. Seguin found music to be the most useful technique. He stated that music helped with exercises and in learning to speak. He said music helped the children learn vowels and consonants and the pitch of speech.

Temple Grandin noted that parents and teachers have reported that they have taught kids to talk through singing. In May, 2016, the television news featured a family that had "discovered" that music would help teach their autistic son to speak. It seems the lessons of the past are easily forgotten.

3. Teach without Speech providing Physical Assistance (Touch).
Seguin adapted to the learning differences by teaching without speech (speech is imitation) and providing physical assistance. He gave an example of teaching body movement with a teacher in front demonstrating the movement and someone assisting the child from behind to make the movement. I found this interesting because I have seen a video from the Higashi School in Japan using this same technique with a class of students with autism. He also gave an example of teaching a child to climb a ladder by physically guiding his arms and legs through the steps.

4. Teach Useful Skills in Proper Environment.
Seguin accommodated the lack of generalization by 1) teaching where the skill is needed; and, 2) teaching useful skills according to their ability. He said the children benefit more from physical training rather than academic training, so they should learn to do useful work and develop good skills and habits.

New Label from Dr. Leo Kanner

Dr. Leo Kanner established the first child psychiatric clinic and published the first textbook on child psychiatry. He is credited with identifying autism as a label for a group of children with similar needs. There were eleven children (8 boys and 3 girls) that were brought to Dr. Kanner's attention from reports from the parents. The children were initially seen when their ages ranged from 2 to 10 years. Dr. Kanner was a diagnostician and created the label, but did not work to help educate them.

In 1943, he published **Autistic Disturbances of Affective Contact** where he identified the main problem as a *"pervasive lack of responsiveness to other people,"* but he also included a description of the children having a positive response to music, excellent rote memory, attention to detail and lack of generalization. He wrote that words could have a specifically literal, inflexible meaning that did not generalize to similar objects or situations, and in some cases, the written language helped with speech. Despite difficulties with communication, some children learned to read, write and spell fairly easily.

Dr. Kanner did a follow-up report in the Journal of Autism and Childhood Schizophrenia in 1971, twenty-eight years after his original identification. These children were born long before the 1975 federal laws regarding special education. Yet, there were a few positive outcomes without the use of special education and we should examine these outcomes to help us find the strategies that were beneficial to their success.

Dr. Kanner reported two positive outcomes with the children who were not institutionalized – Donald T. (case 1) and Frederick W. (case 2). One child, named Herbert B. (case 7), was institutionalized for 23 years, but achieved some success. Just as we can learn effective teaching strategies from Itard and Seguin, we may derive important information from these successful outcomes.

Donald T. (case 1)

At the age of nine, (1942), Donald T. (case 1) was placed on a tenant farm by his parents, who lived about ten miles away. Dr. Kanner visited him three years later, in 1945, and reported that Donald's caretakers were very good at diverting his interests into meaningful use. Donald liked to measure things, so they had him dig a well and report on its depth. He liked to collect dead things, so his caretakers gave him an area for a graveyard where Donald put markers up for the dead animals. When Donald perseverated on counting rows of corn, they directed him to count rows while plowing. In other words, Donald learned by doing useful activities just as Itard and Seguin reported in the 1800's.

In 1970, Don's mother sent a letter of update. She reported that he was 36 years old and living at home. Don received an A.B. degree in French in 1958 and has since worked as a teller in a local bank. The bank was owned by his parents, so we can assume he was given considerable accommodations. His mother reported that he enjoys golf, playing four or five times per week by himself. He was also involved in Kiwanis Club, Jaycees, Investment Club, and Secretary of Presbyterian Sunday School. He drove a car and had a TV, record player and many books in his room. She also noted that he lacked initiative, did not participate in social conversation and showed no interest in the opposite sex.

Frederick Creighton (Wikky) W. (case 2)

Frederick Creighton (Wikky) W. (case 2) (born 1936) attended Devereux School for 23 years. A report from the school in 1962 noted he was able to follow the routine, went on weekend trips into town unaccompanied and made purchases independently. He enjoys music and was a member of the chorus. After leaving Devereux, the family spent a year in Puerto Rico where he enjoyed listening to Spanish language lessons from records. The family moved to Raleigh, N.C. where Creighton attended the County Sheltered Workshop and Vocational Training Center and he enjoyed bowling. He got a job running duplicating (copy) machines and reportedly was doing well.

Herbert B. (case 7)

Herbert B. (Case 7) was born in 1937. He was placed on a farm in Maryland where he followed the farmer around on his chores and learned to cut wood, use the power mower, rake the lawn, set the table and in his spare time, worked jigsaw puzzles. After the farmer died, the widow opened a nursing home for elderly people and Herbert took the old ladies out for walks, brought them trays to their rooms, but never talked.

Secrets Revealed

Drs. Itard and Seguin felt that the abnormalities of sensations were a core deficit and needed to be accommodated in teaching strategies. These symptoms have been ignored or forgotten and were not included in the diagnostic criteria until 2013, but still not identified as an integral part of the disability.

In the 2013 DSM-5, sensory issues were contained under *"Restricted, repetitive patterns of behavior, interests, or activities"*. To receive a diagnosis of ASD (provided in back of book), one only has to meet two of four criteria under restricted, repetitive behaviors. Only one of the criteria mentioned sensory issues stating, *"Hyper-or hypo-reactivity to sensory input or unusual interest in sensory aspects of the environment (e.g. apparent indifference to pain/temperature, adverse response to specific sounds or textures, excessive smelling or touching of objects, visual fascination with lights or movement)."*

This labels behavior related to sensory and perceptual processing, but fails to explain it or relate it to how the child learns. Therefore, sensory issues are not considered a core part of autism, but this is a major mistake. I discuss the abnormalities of sensations and perceptions related to brain function in chapter 6.

Another core deficit identified by Drs. Itard and Seguin are the lack of observation and imitation and lack of generalization. This has never been part of the diagnostic criteria, but the importance is revealed in brain science.

Drs. Itard and Seguin treated children with autism and created teaching strategies. In 1806, Dr. Itard published **The Wild Boy of Aveyron** where he described the deficit of lack of observation and imitation and lack of generalization. He developed a training program of teaching Victor to use practical objects in the environment where they would be used. The child needs to understand the use of objects and not just the labeling of objects. This was teaching "to do" more than "to know" and enabled Victor to attach meaning to objects.

Dr. Seguin expanded on Itard's strategies in 1866 with his publication of **Idiocy and Its Treatment by the Physiological Method**. He added the use of music to teach speech and help with pitch or intonation of speech. Although this approach was ignored or forgotten for a couple centuries, recently this approach has gained attention. I include music as a teaching strategy in the last section of the book.

I found it interesting that Drs. Itard and Seguin did not label the behaviors of autism in a negative manner. They strived to find ways to help the child learn, and responded to strange behaviors as a failure of the teaching strategy. This is in sharp contrast to a focus on strange behaviors in the diagnostic criteria of the 20th and 21st century. We even have an "Aberrant Behavior Checklist" (ABC) that is widely used in assessing the behavior of children with autism. This perspective seems to contribute to our misunderstanding of autism.

Drs. Itard and Seguin's strategy was based on the approach that learning should be fun and not stressful. Dr. Seguin wrote that if we cause stress to the child, then we should remember that we are at fault, and take the child to enjoy music or pleasant exercises. This approach seems to be forgotten or ignored, because today we seem to blame the child for any aberrant behaviors, such as *"not paying attention," "defiant or resistant behavior,"* without any consideration that we may be at fault. Dr. Seguin wrote that teachers should provide pleasure to children, rather than push children to perform for many hours per day, noting that our actions may be causing some of the unwanted behaviors.

Dr. Leo Kanner is credited with identifying a condition he labelled "autism" in 1943. He described these eleven children (8 boys and 3 girls), who were brought to his attention from parents. He did not treat or teach children with autism, but he wrote the first textbook on child psychiatry. He included a description of the children having a positive response to music, excellent rote memory, attention to detail and lack of generalization. This description has never been included in the Diagnostic and Statistical Manual from the American Psychiatric Association. It is important information that has been ignored.

Twenty-eight years after Dr. Kanner's identification, in 1971, he did a follow-up report that found two positive outcomes. This was before the 1975 federal laws regarding special education. Kanner's cases of Herbert and Donald illustrate the success of teaching to strengths and learning to do chores. This is teaching "to do" rather than "to know." The skills are sometimes structured with counting or measuring, giving meaning from the child's perspective or strengths. The teaching strategies included turning the child's interests into meaningful activities. These teaching strategies are some of the forgotten secrets of autism.

The next chapter will discuss how our attitudes and treatment of the disabled changed over time as a result of social and political influences.

Chapter 2

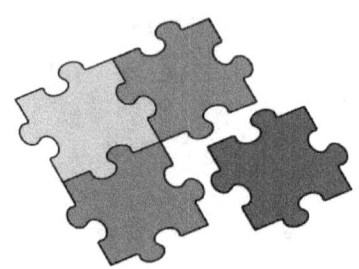

The Pendulum Swings

"Everybody is a genius. But if you judge a fish by its ability to climb a tree, it will live its whole life believing that it is stupid." Albert Einstein

In the 1880's there was a large influx of immigrants coming into the United States and the nation's leaders were concerned about unwanted immigrants, because they wanted to create a good citizenry. They wanted people who would contribute to the economy and not become a drain upon it. In 1882, Congress passed the Undesirables Act that prevented convicts, paupers, the insane, and idiots from entering the U.S. The prevailing thought was that those with mental deficiency -- now mainly referred to as "feebleminded" -- had bad genes and were a threat to society.

In 1892, Ellis Island, located in New York Harbor near the Statue of Liberty, opened as a federal immigration site. The water surrounding the island was too shallow for transatlantic ships, so they docked in Manhattan. American citizens and first and second-class passengers were allowed to enter the country after a brief inspection. Third-class or steerage passengers were loaded onto barges and taken to Ellis Island. Upon arrival, immigrants were paraded before a series of medical officers for inspection. Those immigrants who seemed to have physical or mental deficiencies were taken away for additional screening. Any signs of contagious disease, physical deformities, feeblemindedness or insanity could result in denied entrance, based on the premise that they were likely to become a burden on the state.

Psychiatrists also judged children and adult citizens who lived in the United States, to determine who might be blind, deaf, epileptic, poor, or prone to criminal behaviors, have strange behaviors or were slow to learn. Any behavior outside of what was considered "good citizenry" was open to judgment by a psychiatrist for a label of "feeblemindedness", resulting in removal from their families and placement in an institution. Society accepted the power and authority of a group of psychiatrists to label and treat a large segment of the population, who could not protest any action against them.

When psychiatrists claimed they were helping society by removing the unwanted, state governments were convinced to help fund the institutions, thus promoting the value and respect of the specialty of psychiatry. Once a "cause" of the problems of society was promulgated and accepted, then the treatment that followed was easily justified. We segregated the unwanted from society and promoted sterilization, so they could not reproduce the bad genes.

Families were made to feel shame in having a mentally or physically disabled child, and they were pressured to place them in an institution. Once the psychiatrists had defined their specialty, giving them authority and control over the population in institutions, a parent was unable to simply remove their child from the institution, but had to request permission from the psychiatrist, who required families to post bonds of $1000 or more. Since many families were unable to afford such an amount, psychiatrists had effectively taken away the authority of the parent. Tens of thousands of people, who died in state institutions, were buried in graves marked only by numbers. People believed at the time that having names on the grave markers would be shameful to the families of the deceased.

Creation of Mental Testing

From 1906 to 1918, Henry Goddard (1866-1957) was the Director of Research at the Vineland Training School for Feebleminded in Vineland, New Jersey. He had a Master's degree in mathematics and a Doctorate in psychology. Goddard was searching for a way to diagnose the feebleminded and he came upon the French test for slow learners, called the Simon-Binet Scale, published in 1905.

Why was this test developed? In 1904, the French Ministry of Education asked Alfred Binet (1857-1911), a French psychologist, to devise a method that would determine which students did not learn effectively from regular classroom instruction, so they could be given more individualized instruction in separate classes.

Alfred Binet and Theodore Simon (1872-1961), a medical student, developed the Simon-Binet scale that consisted of thirty tasks of increasing difficulty. Some of the tasks required students to point to various body parts, repeat simple sentences and to define some everyday words. More difficult tasks included finding the differences between pairs of things and when given three words, the student needed to make a sentence including these words. The most difficult tasks revealed abstract thinking. They discovered that certain tasks typical students could pass, but a few students could not.

The test result was interpreted as a mental age compared to the chronological age. For example, a typical eight year old who could pass all the tasks for that age, would score an eight, while another eight year old might pass tasks that a typical five year old could pass and he would score a five.

The test was designed to be given individually, as this would enable the tester to observe the strengths and weaknesses of the individual learner. Giving a test to a group does not allow one to observe the individual, and discover how they think and how to find ways to help that person learn. The Simon-Binet test was published in 1905.

In 1908 Goddard translated the test into English and administered it to the children at Vineland. He validated his results by comparing them to what the teachers had to say about the students. (Note: Using someone's opinion to validate a test is not science-based!) Goddard took a giant leap and claimed the test measured a mental ability called intelligence that was not defined.

He created a labeling method to be used with the mental test. He divided the feebleminded into three classes: 1) Idiots have deeply defective mental development that does not exceed a mental age of about two years; 2) Imbeciles whose mental development does not exceed a mental age of about seven years; and 3) Morons whose mental development does not exceed a mental age of about twelve years. Moron comes from the Greek word meaning "foolish."

This labeling system changed the purpose of the test from helping children obtain extra instruction, to conveying the idea that some children cannot learn beyond a certain age. It is a judgment of the value of another human being, and it is no surprise that many parents did not appreciate having their children judged and labeled.

In 1910, Goddard, a psychologist, managed to convince the psychiatrists of the Association of Medical Officers of American Institutions for Feeble-minded Persons (later known as the AAMR – American Association for the Mentally Retarded) to adopt a mental test as a means of establishing a diagnosis for the feebleminded. Since this seemed more scientific than a physical description, it was readily accepted. It also supported the prevailing belief that the feebleminded were a threat to our goal to establish a good citizenry. Although it helped psychiatrists with a labeling system, it also gave Goddard a professional boost and would create a major testing industry that aligned psychology with education.

Since Goddard worked in Vineland, New Jersey, he was able to sell his IQ method to the state government. In 1911, the IQ test became part of the law in New Jersey requiring special education classes for students who scored 3 years below their chronological age. This would create a new niche for psychologists to test school children and they would become a significant part of the public school system.

Goddard believed that intelligence was hereditary and feeblemindedness was the cause of all of society's problems. He wanted to prove his belief in bad genes as the cause of feeblemindedness. He hired "field workers" to track relatives of children in the Vineland school. Their goal was to document the family history in order to demonstrate the laws of inheritance. One of these field workers, Elizabeth Kite, reported to Goddard that she had evidence tracing back six generations of a child in Vineland given a pseudonym of Deborah (real name Emma Wolverton).

Kite demonstrated two branches of the family – one was the good side of the family with children becoming professionals and associated with the best families, and the second was the bad side with children becoming social burdens because of illegitimate births, alcoholism, criminals, prostitutes and paupers. Goddard invented the family name "*Kallikak*" by combining Greek root meanings for "*good*" and "*bad*".

Martin Kallikak, Sr. was a Revolutionary War Hero who fathered a son, Martin Kallikak, Jr. with a feebleminded bar maid. Despite this indiscretion, Martin, Sr. was married to a respectable woman from a good family. The descendants from the bar maid were the bad side of the family and the descendants of the upper class woman were only successful individuals of normal intelligence. To Goddard the good side suggested the control group and the bad side demonstrated the "bad genes" that are passed down resulting in social problems.

In 1912, Goddard published *The Kallikak Family: A study in the Heredity of Feeble-Mindedness.* In 1927, the study was introduced as evidence in a Supreme Court case Buck v. Bell that legalized involuntary sterilization of "moral defectives" (anyone deemed to be feebleminded). After the U.S. Supreme Court decision, the number of sterilizations increased. This was a situation where a professional wanted to promote their personal belief and he presented one family history in an attempt to "prove" that belief. This is not a scientific study and it demonstrates how we are often willing to accept a professional's statement as true, simply because it supports what we want to believe.

Henry Goddard established a testing program on third class immigrants at Ellis Island in 1913. His testing found an estimated 80% of immigrants feebleminded, resulting in a sudden increase in deportations. Goddard targeted Jews, Italians, Russians and Hungarians. The testing only proved what he already believed about immigrants from the lower class.

Madison Grant (1865-1937), a lawyer, was one of the founders of the American Eugenics Society (AES) established in 1926. Eugenics comes from the Greek words for "good" and "origin" to connote "good birth," or "well born." Grant published *The Passing of the Great Race* in 1916, wherein he stated *"The laws of nature require the obliteration of the unfit, and human life is valuable only when it is of use to the community."* I was surprised when I read about the widespread support and acceptance of the eugenics movement in the United States. Members and advisors to the eugenics society were from elite universities in the country and included some of the best psychologists, psychiatrists, doctors and scientists. Part of the justification for eugenics was based on the burden of high costs incurred to care for these defectives.

Robert Whitaker writes in *Mad in America* that the media and medical journals supported the sterilization of mental defectives and over fifty percent of Americans favored the practice stating, *"By the end of 1945,*

29

45,127 Americans had been sterilized." The eventual goal of eugenics was to create a superior human race.

The eugenics movement took hold in Germany in the 1930's. After World War I, Germany lay in ruins and many of its healthy men had died. Because of the poor economy and concern over paying for the cost of care for mental defectives, the eugenics movement from the United States took hold in Germany. In 1925, Adolph Hitler published **Mein Kampf** that promoted eugenics as the science needed to rebuild the nation. Adolph Hitler took control of the government in 1933 and he would take this idea to the extreme by killing all inferiors, including Jews, elderly, sick and retarded children and adults. In 1934, the Kallikak book was published in Nazi Germany.

Nazi Germany targeted people with disabilities and the elderly as a drain on public resources. They were referred to as *"useless eaters."* Persons with disabilities – over 200,000 – were the first victims of the Holocaust, but what you hear about Nazi Germany is the killing of Jews, because that distances America from the World War II atrocities.

Most people are aware of the killings in Nazi Germany with the Holocaust, but don't seem to realize the idea of bad genes and removing these people from society began in the United States. We justified our use of sterilization and turned a blind-eye to the abuse and neglect in the institutions resulting in the death of thousands of people left in unmarked graves.

Goddard was a busy man effectively promoting his ideas through the use of his intelligence test as 1) beneficial to psychiatrists to remove anyone deemed unworthy to live in society; 2) beneficial to public schools for managing large numbers of children; 3) preventing the unwanted from immigrating into the country; 4) determining job tracks for military in WWI; 5) writing a book on the Kallikak family to support his beliefs in eugenics, that was used in the courts to promote sterilization as a means of controlling bad genes from being passed to the next generation; 6) creating terminology to make his ideas seem science-based and professional; and, 7) building a testing empire and a specialty for psychology.

Testing used to Support Common Belief in U.S

Other psychologists jumped on the bandwagon to help promote testing, as well as promoting their personal and professional agendas. Lewis Madison Terman (1877-1956), American psychologist, joined the faculty of Stanford University in 1910 as professor of educational psychology. He revised the Simon-Binet scale and published the Stanford Binet test in 1916. He served as chairman of the psychology department from 1922-1945.

Terman adopted the scoring method of dividing mental age by chronological age and multiplying by 100 to achieve an intelligence quotient or IQ score. It is called a "quotient," because it is achieved by dividing by chronological age. He defined intelligence as "the ability to carry on abstract thinking" (1921 Journal of Educational Psychology).

Terman believed IQ was inherited and was the best predictor of success in life. Terman was involved in the first mass administration of the IQ test on 1.7 million soldiers during World War I, to determine the appropriate job track (separate officers). After the war, Terman and colleagues promoted the IQ test in American schools to determine the appropriate job-track. In other words, how you performed on a test as a child or young adult (military) would determine what opportunities would be available for you. It would not matter how hard you worked, you would be blocked from changing this future direction set for you by a test.

Despite Binet's warnings, psychologists in America used the mental test to promote the perspective that mentally retarded had a genetic condition that made them a menace to society. It was an easy sell, because most people in society already believed in the unworthiness of individuals with mental deficiencies. The IQ test simply provided the justification for the identification of the unfortunates to be segregated in state institutions. Since the problem was identified as genetic, the "solution" became sterilization to prevent future generations of the unwanted. There was no intention of helping children learn.

Many people with mental defects have physical differences and this was emphasized so people would become fearful of those with physical defects, who were to be seen as a menace to society. The fear of people with physical deformities has long been popular in the media. *The Hunchback of Notre Dame* was a French novel published by Victor Hugo in 1831 and

Frankenstein was a novel by English author Mary Shelley, first published in 1818 and then published in France in 1823. This depiction of disabled to be feared continued into the 20th century with the *Wolfman*, a 1941 American film.

Testing Changes Organization of Public Schools

Goddard had already sold the idea of IQ testing to psychiatrists, as a means of labeling people to justify their removal to the institutions that the psychiatrists directed. The next step was to sell it to the public school system. The timing was perfect. In the 1920's schools in the United States were struggling with a sudden large increase in the number of students. This was due to three factors: 1) legally mandating education that required young people to attend school; 2) large influx of foreign speaking immigrants; and, 3) handling students who could not keep up with other students.

Goddard, Terman and others trumpeted the IQ test that would give a single number as a means of helping the schools to rank and separate students. This would be a major change in the organization of the schools. It had not been necessary to separate children previously, so children of different ages were within the same classroom and proceeding at their own pace. Now children could be separated into classes by chronological age (a new idea), and those that could not keep up could be placed in separate classes. With the IQ test, if a child scored less than his chronological age, it justified removal from the class and placement into a special class. But rather than viewing the special class as a method of helping children learn, it became associated with the idea that the children had been removed from the class, because they could not learn.

The IQ classification system used mental testing to determine a specific educational category and class placement based on assumptions about the capabilities of students. The terms used were: 1) Educable Mental Retardation (EMR) for IQ range of 50-75; 2) Trainable Mental Retardation (TMR) for IQ range of 25-50; and 3) Severe and Profound Mental Retardation (SPMR) for IQ below 25. Most children with mental retardation would be in the mild range of 50-75.

Charles Hart in his 1989 book, *Without Reason*, wrote how he took the school system to due process in order to get language therapy for his autistic son. The school argued that his son was mentally retarded and would not benefit from the therapy – reflecting the perspective of educators during the 20th Century. Although the school technically "lost," they were only required to give a mere two hours of therapy a week.

The original purpose of the test to help children with extra instruction was discarded, when American psychologists attempted to promote the specialty of psychology. They claimed that mental retardation was hereditary, a social problem, and could not be improved by education. Once people accepted this idea of giving someone a number from a test to determine their success in life and the quality of an individual, it became a self-fulfilling prophecy.

The Pendulum Swings

The Great Depression (1929-1939) of the United States created changing social conditions and new experiences for people that slowly created a new way of thinking. Many people were out of work and could not find work. With the depression, previously employed men were standing in "bread lines" and fighting poverty. Standing in long lines to obtain food helped people understand that anyone could be vulnerable and need help. Suddenly, the idea that the problems in society were due to bad genes didn't make as much sense.

The depression resulted in overcrowding in the institutions and long waiting lists for admittance. As a result, psychiatrists started releasing those with mild retardation. In 1941 after the bombing of Pearl Harbor, America mobilized for war. Superintendents of the institutions were surprised when contacted by military recruitment services for information about former residents.

The American Association on Mental Deficiency (AAMD) response was that most people with mental deficiency would not be able to adjust to military duties. They advocated training them for menial jobs that would enable more able people to serve in the military. But the social condition of war resulted in great demands for recruitment that made careful selection impossible. At the beginning of U.S. involvement, thousands of men were being inducted every day. Many runaways and released residents from the institutions were succeeding in enlisting in the armed services.

Military psychologists said IQ was not meaningful as a determinant of a person's ability to serve. The military was not interested in labels. They needed to find a way for feebleminded men to be useful. This resulted in many people previously labeled and institutionalized demonstrating that they could adapt, thus transforming their social status. This was a surprise to many professionals who had spent a lifetime labeling and treating the mental defectives and would result in a need to reformulate their definitions of mental deficiency.

The return of disabled veterans from World War II also changed attitudes. Society felt an obligation to treat those men and women who had fought for our freedoms. Some mental defectives had demonstrated that they could adapt to real-life situations and this promulgated the perspective that those with disabilities simply needed opportunities. The war had revealed that many social problems were the result of those with normal intelligence, which would challenge the perspective that social problems were caused by those with low intelligence.

Parents of Disabled Push for Social Change

After World War II (1939-1945), doctors continued to encourage parents to institutionalize their children with mental retardation, warning that the extraordinary needs of such a child would adversely affect the marriage and other children in the family. This was an example of professionals who found another excuse - that was more acceptable to the public – in order to do what they intended to do anyway. Despite such dire advice, some prominent parents began to speak out against the attitude of shame associated with having a child with mental retardation.

Attitudes in society were slow to change. President Franklin Delano Roosevelt was an adult victim of polio, and went to great lengths to hide his disability from the public, but his personal experience created empathy for the disabled and he established the March of Dimes in 1938. Other charity organizations followed with the United Cerebral Palsy started in 1949 and the League for Muscular Dystrophy in 1950.

In 1950, Pearl Buck published *The Child Who Never Grew*, portraying her daughter, Carol, as an innocent child with mental retardation. In 1953, Dale Evans and Roy Rogers, a well-known acting family, spoke out about their mentally retarded child. Dale Evans published a book *Angel*

Unaware about her daughter, Robin, who died at the age of two. The Kennedy family finally acknowledged the existence of Rose Marie "Rosie" Kennedy (1918-2005), when John F. Kennedy was President of the United States. Edward Shorter wrote in *The Kennedy Family and the Story of Mental Retardation* that Rosemary's mother did not confide in her friends and that she pretended Rosie was normal, with relatives beyond the immediate family knowing nothing of Rosemary's condition. But Eunice Kennedy Shriver published an article in 1962 with the Saturday Evening Post revealing the true story of Rosemary's condition.

In 1948, parents of mentally retarded children began forming support groups and advocating for acceptance, education and inclusion into their communities. This would not only change the opportunities for disabled children, but it would begin to redefine the concept of the normal family. The groups argued that their disabled children deserved the same care and services the community gave to normal families. In 1950, the National Association for Retarded Children (NARC) was established.

The 1950's culture emphasized the ideal family life as portrayed on television with *Leave it to Beaver* and *Father Knows Best.* The perspective that mentally retarded were a threat to society was replaced by the fear mental retardation could destroy the idealized family. As late as 1989, this perspective continued in the medical community. My husband, Jerry and I went to a psychiatrist at the recommendation of a school psychologist to help us adjust to having a disabled child. This psychiatrist told us that most families divorce as a result of having a disabled child. Her pessimistic attitude was not helpful and we decided not to see her again. Our marriage survived.

There were several factors to overcome in order for special education to become available: 1) Educators felt only children deemed educable should go to school and not those with IQ's less than 50; 2) There were few trained teachers or even educational programs for training teachers; 3) Funding was a challenge for providing an education that was deemed to have questionable value.

By the 1970's, parent groups were incorporating the perspective of the civil rights movement. The family groups argued that disabilities were caused by lack of opportunity, rather than bad genes. Children with mental retardation were disabled by society and the attitudes toward them. The problem was environmental, and the solution would be to provide greater equality and access to public education and community services. Even the most severely disabled were assumed capable of leading quality lives in society. Families fought for their disabled children to have an education to prepare them to take their place in society. It was argued that many aberrant behaviors were caused by labeling and being in institutions.

A new theory developed called *"normalization,"* where children should be educated in regular classes and have access to the community. It was believed that if disabled children were educated with typical peers, they would learn proper social skills. Some professionals argued that when children are labeled and placed in separate classrooms, they show more behaviors related to disabilities, and if children are educated with typical peers then they become "normal".

Federal Government takes Control of Special Education

When John F. Kennedy was president (1960-1963), he promulgated federal law to provide research and services for mental retardation through the President's Panel on Mental Retardation. It was his sister, Eunice Kennedy Shriver, who was the driving force behind this legislation. The changes shifted funding from the state institutions to the National Institute on Child Health and Human Development (NICHHD). This separated monies from mental illness, and also supported research on mental retardation. Monies were provided to University associated hospitals to establish teaching services where mental retardation specialists would help with diagnosis and treatment. This resulted in dozens of research labs at university hospitals.

After the Kennedy administration started the funding for mental retardation, other disability groups demanded the same. When new legislation was introduced to Congress in 1970, the term *"developmental disabilities"* was introduced. The question became, *"Who should be considered developmentally disabled?"* This was a political issue. Some wanted all children included, even the most severely handicapped, who were typically not included in receiving social services. President Nixon (1969-1974) opposed the bill because of the cost, and he wanted to restrict funding to research and not services, but the moral argument forced him to sign the bill, since politicians do not wish to be perceived as uncaring.

The Developmental Disabilities Services and Facilities Act of 1970 included those with mental retardation, and epilepsy and other conditions associated with mental retardation. Autism was considered a mental illness – a form of schizophrenia – so it was not included. Mrs. Shriver had separated funding for mental retardation and mental illness, and the creators of this bill did not want to incur the anger of psychiatrists with the National Institute for Mental Health.

Autism was not included in the 1970 Developmental Disabilities and Facilities Act, so funding for this disability was scarce. Psychiatrists came under pressure to change the description of autism from a form of schizophrenia to a pervasive developmental disability (PDD) in 1980 to gain access to government funding. This change came from politics – not any science – and the authority and power of psychiatrists was diminishing.

In 1975, The Individuals with Disabilities Education Act (IDEA) was passed that provided for education for all disabled children in the *"least restrictive environment."* The bill not only required public schools to educate children with disabilities but also gave legal grounds for parents to insist children with disabilities should be included in regular classrooms. The theory of normalization was prevalent in this legislation that would change the organization of public school special education. Educators were not ready to accept this new ideology, because they were taught the IQ test would determine school placement and the type of education. It would take a couple of decades – and numerous lawsuits – to force public schools to comply with this belief.

This legislation set a precedent for parents of disabled children to be more involved in the decision of how education would be provided to their children. Some parents would use the law to demand services, such as speech and language therapy, occupational therapy, and behavioral therapy. The law also stated no discussion of cost was allowed during the educational planning process for a disabled child, but this created a problem for the interactions between parents and educators. Educators have to work within a budget and some costs for educating children with disabilities skyrocketed. Since educators could not state that the problem of providing services was lack of money, they would argue that the service was not needed. This often resulted in considerable conflicts between educators and parents.

Federal spending on research and education for children with disabilities soared to almost 8 billion dollars in 1985. This was a reflection of the new attitude of providing compensation for previous injustices. The civil rights movement coincided with the fight for disabled children. They advocated the same ideas - that everyone was entitled to the same opportunities and quality of life and deserved compensation for past injustices.

This perspective spread throughout the country. There was little objection to increased government control and increased spending, since it was providing benefits for people deserving assistance and compensation. Medicaid was started and there seemed to be no limit to the availability of monies.

The federal laws were well intended to try to change the perception of disabled children and increase their participation in the community, but the law went too far by stating children with disabilities should be educated in the same classrooms with more able students. An IQ test simply measures academic performance and there will always be some above average and some below average.

We all have different abilities even within academics – some shine in mathematics or foreign languages (and I certainly don't in either field!!). Some people will shine in the area of music, dance, art or sports. All areas can be measured and result in a bell curve, where there are some who are average, some above average, and some below average. The problem was created when we perceived a test as a reflection of the worth of a human being, when it was merely intended to identify and provide extra assistance to those who are not as strong academically. The goal is not to "cure" mental retardation or ignore the below average performance in academics, but to help these children find their strengths to becoming more independent and self-reliant as adults.

Attempts to Raise Intelligence

If you don't know history, you are very apt to repeat the mistakes of the past. The field of mental retardation continues to repeat past mistakes. Drs. Itard and Seguin believed mental retardation could be cured with *"education of the senses."* Many institutions became training centers, but when the cure did not occur, some training schools became merely custodial institutions.

The eugenics movement promoted the idea that mental retardation was inherited and could not be cured, so professionals promoted the belief that mental retardation presented a menace to society. Sterilization was instituted to prevent future generations of people with mental retardation.

When the pendulum swung back to the idea that disabilities were caused by the environment, various therapies were promoted to cure mental retardation. One group believed that mental retardation was caused by a lack of opportunities of interaction between children and parents. Another group, the behaviorists, believed that the parents of children with mental retardation caused it by giving the wrong *"reinforcements"* for various behaviors. In other words, blame the parents!

Some professionals want to believe they can cure mental retardation and will convince themselves that they can. Herman H. Spitz authored **The Raising of Intelligence: A selected History of Attempts to Raise Retarded Intelligence,** and he wrote that John Throne and his colleagues at the University of Kansas claimed in the 1970's that mental retardation could be reversed with behavioral training. They taught children to perform well on the twelve subtests of the Wechsler Intelligence Scale for Children as well as on the Picture Peabody test. Although they claimed retarded children could reach normal intelligence, there has been a failure to replicate the studies.

Herman Spitz also reported that the Milwaukee Project (Herber and colleagues 1972) was widely touted for its claim that an enriched environment for disadvantaged children can increase IQ scores an average of 33 points. The program provided intense one-to-one interaction and parent training. It was apparently more wishful thinking and lacked proper scientific study. Some professionals seem to think it is a race for a cure and they become more focused on competition with other professionals and different teaching strategies, rather than seeking the best way to help children with disabilities learn.

Chapter 4 on *Applied Behavior Analysis* discusses the study in 1987 by behaviorist Ivar Lovaas that is often cited as the scientific basis for this therapy for children with autism. He cites the raising of intelligence as a measure for "recovery" of some students in his study. Unfortunately, there are still researchers today, who think they can cure mental retardation and use IQ scores as outcome measures.

The inability to raise intelligence is unrelated to the need to give all mentally retarded individuals an appropriate education in order for them to reach their potential. Low intelligence is no barrier to individuals becoming functioning members of society.

The Struggle to Define Mental Retardation

The 1961 AAMD (American Association on Mental Deficiency) established the term *"mental retardation"* to replace the previous terms of *"idiocy"* or *"feeblemindedness."* Changing labels is common practice that ensures political correctness and reflects social philosophy. In 2010, President Obama changed the term mental retardation to *"intellectual disabilities."*

The 1961 American Association of Mental Retardation (AAMR) manual was the first to use test scores and required a score greater than one standard deviation below the mean (less than 85). This resulted in a large number of children (16%) who would qualify for special education services and this would require significant funding.

The 1973 AAMR manual changed the cut-off for mental retardation from 85 to 70, reducing the number of children diagnosed from 16% to approximately 2.2%. This was the definition included in the Education for All Handicapped Children Act of 1975 (IDEA, PL94-142) that was intended to give all disabled children access to an education. Therefore, the definition of mental retardation was altered for political purposes, because it would be too expensive to serve so many children.

Most children identified as mentally retarded are in the mild range (70-85). Some children can receive a low score, but adapt well to adult life, but others require more help. The challenge was to identify the children with mild mental retardation, who would benefit from special education. Professionals needed more than a number on a test to determine who was eligible for special education.

In an attempt to more clearly define those children who require special education, the 1977 AAMR manual allowed the diagnosis of mental retardation for children with IQ's up to ten points (80) above the 70 cutoff, if they also showed marked deficits in adaptive behavior that was described as *"The effectiveness or degree with which the individual meets the standards of personal independence and social responsibility expected of his age and cultural grouping."*

The 1992 definition from the AAMR reads: *"Mental retardation refers to substantial limitations in <u>present functioning</u>. It is characterized by significantly sub average intellectual functioning, existing concurrently with related limitations in two or more of the following applicable adaptive skill areas: communication, self-care, home living, social skills, community use, self-direction, health and safety, functional academics, leisure and work."* The addition of *"present functioning"* in the 1992 definition conveyed the belief in curing mental retardation with education. This represented the social perspective that changed the description of mental retardation from a hereditary cause to an environmental cause. The pendulum had swung from Seguin in the 1800's claiming he could cure mental retardation to bad genes in the 1900's then back to curing mental retardation by education in the 1950's to 1970's.

In 2002, the AAMR changed *"hereditary effects"* on mental retardation to *"intergenerational effects"* of environmental influences that can be prevented or reversed through education. This was not a report of results from science, but simply changing social perspective of mental retardation being from bad genes to a condition that can be cured or reversed.

The AAMR also changed the definition from differentiated levels of mental retardation as mild, moderate, severe and profound to specifying levels of support. It specified <u>intermittent needs</u> are episodic in nature and do not always require support; <u>limited needs</u> are consistent over time but limited in intensity<u>; extensive needs</u> are long-term and serious; and <u>pervasive needs</u> are constant and intense throughout life. This was a new concept in mental retardation that the primary purpose of diagnosis is intervention planning. This reflects the changing social and political climate and ignores science.

There is considerable controversy over these attempts to define mental retardation. A good book from 2006 about this controversy is "**What is Mental Retardation? Ideas for an Evolving Disability in the 21**[st]

41

Century, by editors Switzky and Greenspan. We seem to have strayed from the idea of mental testing to help us teach children, to an assumption that a score on a test somehow reflects "intelligence." When a definition is based on a false assumption, then perhaps one should consider a new premise. With the advancement of brain science, we know that thinking skills reflect brain function, and a lack of connections in the brain change thinking and learning abilities.

Brain connections are required for processing information and learning. In 2007, Science Daily reported that research has demonstrated the brain requires connections (primarily involving areas in the frontal and parietal lobes) to process information. These areas include those related to attention, memory and language. Research scientists Richard J. Haier and Rex E. Jung reviewed 37 imaging studies in the Journal of Behavioral and Brain Sciences and found that intelligence is related to how efficiently information travels through the brain.

Definitions change over time, often a reflection of changing social perspectives. I have described how the pendulum has swung from a belief in curing mental retardation to a belief in the menace of mental retardation that could not be corrected, back to a belief that we can cure mental retardation with school or behavior therapy. When we don't know history, we are prone to repeating the mistakes of the past, often basing our assumptions on a false premise. We no longer need to rely on a score from a mental test to determine an individual's ability to process information. It is time to take a new direction to helping children with autism learn by basing teaching strategies on brain science.

Mental Retardation in Autism

In 2008, the Center for Disease Control (CDC) reported 38% of children with autism have mental retardation, with 24% borderline. Autism is more frequent in boys than girls (4:1), but a higher proportion (48%) of autistic females have mental retardation. Since the CDC has been measuring prevalence rates of autism with co-occurring mental retardation, the rates of individuals who do not have MR has been rising. This is not surprising, since higher functioning individuals (Asperger Syndrome) were added to the diagnostic category in 1994. As more high functioning children are included under the same label, then the percentage of those with mental retardation will decrease.

The educational system relies primarily on normal development and ability to perform academic skills. Normal IQ scores have been historically associated with the ability to learn life skills easily and without specific teaching. Life skills include such activities as chores, dressing, shopping, laundry, crossing the street, accessing public transportation and public places. These are not skills typically taught in school.

It was assumed that children who were not mentally retarded would naturally learn life skills. The diagnostic criteria for Asperger's Syndrome that was added in 1994 stated, *"In contrast to Autistic Disorder, there are no clinically significant delays in language. In addition there are no clinically significant delays in cognitive development or in the development of age-appropriate self-help skills, adaptive behavior, and curiosity about the environment in childhood."* They were wrong.

Recent studies have revealed the surprising outcome that young adults with autism, and normal scores on IQ tests, have not learned life skills that enable them to reach independence and self-sufficiency as adults. In 2007, Ami Kline and associates published a study with a conclusion that instruction in life skills should be intensified as children with autism get older. They recommend that life skill instruction should be a priority.

A 2007 study by S. Williams White and colleagues concluded that educating children with autism in the regular classroom does not meet their needs for life skills. While most children with Asperger's Syndrome can adjust to a regular classroom and handle the academic demands, the curriculum does not address their needs for life skills training. Thus, education for ALL children with autism has gone awry.

Secrets Revealed

IQ is a number manipulated over the years to serve different purposes. It was originally developed to help children who could not learn at the same pace as their peers. It was used as a "scientific" means of identifying children and adults that were removed from society and placed in institutions.

During WWI, the IQ test was used to determine job tracks for people entering the military, but during WWII military psychologists determined that the IQ score was not useful to determine a person's ability to serve. Many people previously removed from society were now serving in the U.S. military. This would result in institutional psychiatrists and psychologists having to alter their perspectives and admission criteria.

After WWII, the pendulum swung back to the belief in educating children with disabilities. The definition of mental retardation was changed several times based on social and political needs. The determination of mental retardation (IQ score) was adjusted to prevent too many children from being identified as eligible for special education, as this would cost the government too much money. It was also adjusted based on the belief in "bad genes" changing to a belief in curing intelligence through education.

Dr. Ramachandran in **The Tell-Tale Brain** (2011) wrote that use of IQ scores would be analogous to saying that general health is a heritable trait and can be measured as a single number – age. He stated that any medical student who associated general health with a single number, such as age, would never be allowed to become a medical doctor. He writes: *"Yet whole careers in psychology and political movements have been built on the equally absurd belief in single measurable general intelligence."* This ridiculous idea has become so entrenched in our society that the masses regard it as the truth.

Education for children with autism should not be based on intelligence scores. When higher functioning children were added to the autism label, there was the expectation that they did not need to be taught life skills, because we don't normally teach children these skills in the classroom. Educators have discovered that children with autism, who do not have mental retardation, have not learned life skills in the regular classroom that will enable them to become independent adults. An IQ score does not ensure the individual will be able to learn life skills as neurotypical (NT) children can. We now know that all children with autism require life skills training and this is not identified by a number on a test and can't be obtained in the regular classroom.

Since federal law requires the education of disabled children in the regular classroom, unless withdrawal is justified by the school, changing an entrenched policy is extremely difficult. As we have seen, it often requires numerous lawsuits to force a change in a belief system.

The focus on IQ scores has distracted us from the real needs of children with autism. Dr. Kanner and other professionals promoted the idea of the child with hidden intelligence, so we searched to treat the child to reveal this intelligence and make them normal. In 1994, Asperger's Syndrome was added resulting in children without mental retardation being included as autistic.

In 2013, the diagnostic criteria became a spectrum by combining different pervasive developmental disabilities under one label. It seems more appropriate to identify the specific learning needs of children with autism and creating teaching strategies that can be individualized to the children, rather than trying to teach to this unknown trait called "intelligence."

Intelligence is related to how fast information is processed in the brain. Brain science now teaches us how children learn differently based on the structure and function of the brain. It is time to focus on teaching strategies for children with disabilities that accommodate the differences in brain structure and function.

The next chapter will discuss changing psychiatric labels and psychiatric treatments of children with autism.

Chapter 3

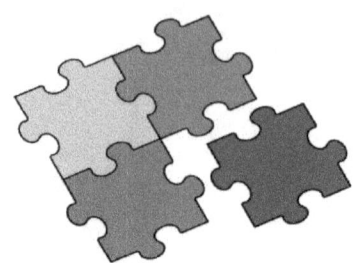

Psychiatric Labels and Treatments

"Most of the greatest evils that man has inflicted upon man have come through people feeling quite certain about something which, in fact, was false." Bertrand Russell

Dr. Leo Kanner (pronounced Conner; 1894-1981) was promoting a new specialty called child psychiatry. Dr. Kanner was born in Austria and educated in Berlin, Germany. He received his M.D. from the University of Berlin in 1921, and emigrated to the U.S. in 1924, to work at Yankton State Hospital (a mental hospital) in Yankton, South Dakota. Although he was trained as a cardiologist, he switched to psychiatry when he came to the United States.

In 1928, Dr. Kanner went to Johns Hopkins in Baltimore, Maryland where he established the first child psychiatric clinic. He published the first textbook on child psychiatry in 1935 and he was a well-respected person of authority in the area of child psychiatry.

In 1938, Kanner was introduced to a 5 year old, named Donald T., when Donald's father, a lawyer, wrote an extensive letter to Dr. Kanner documenting his son's strange behaviors. Donald was brought to Baltimore by his parents to stay for two weeks at the Harriet Lane Home (part of Johns Hopkins) to be evaluated by Dr. Kanner and his staff.

Dr. Kanner was baffled by Donald's strange behaviors that he had never seen before, but over the next four years more parents contacted Dr. Kanner regarding their children, who all had similar behaviors. Dr. Kanner documented eleven cases in his 1943 publication *"Autistic Disturbance of*

Affective Contact." Later, he changed the label to *"early infantile autism"* to indicate that it was present in early childhood.

Kanner tried to walk a thin line with regards to mental retardation, perhaps because some of the parents were psychiatrists, and all were well educated. Several of the children had been diagnosed as idiots or imbeciles, one resided in a state school for the feebleminded and two had been labeled schizophrenic. Kanner stated he was unable to test the children with intelligence tests, because of their limited verbal ability. Kanner concluded that *"they are all unquestionably endowed with good cognitive potentialities."* This was wishful thinking on Kanner's part, but because he was considered the authority on the disorder, this perspective would continue and contribute to the belief in a hidden intelligence. This was a time in history where mental retardation was considered shameful and related to "bad genes," so Kanner would not want to place such a label on children whose parents are professionals. He stated *"It is not easy to evaluate the fact that all of our patients have come of highly intelligent parents."*

Kanner was careful in his wording of the cause of autism. He noted there were very few affectionate mothers and fathers of autistic children, as they were preoccupied with professions and had limited interest in people. He stated the marriages were *"rather cold and formal affairs."* He was unable to determine to what extent the parental behavior contributed to the child's condition.

Bettelheim and Refrigerator Mother

Blaming parents for the cause of autism was highly touted by Bruno Bettelheim, (1903-1990). He was Austrian born and claimed he spent 11 months as a prisoner in Dachau and Buchenwald concentration camps from 1938-1939. He somehow gained release from the concentration camp to come to New York in 1939. He moved to Chicago and became a U.S. citizen in 1944. Although he was an art historian, he became professor of psychology at the University of Chicago from 1944 until his retirement in 1973. He studied Freud, psychoanalysis and emotionally disturbed children.

Bettelheim served as director of the Orthogenic School for disturbed children in Chicago. "Orthogenic" means relating to the treatment or correction of mental and emotional abnormalities in children. It was Bettelheim who promoted the widespread acceptance of the *"refrigerator mother*" theory to the public and medical establishment in the 1950's and 1960's. This theory blamed the mother for causing autism, because she was cold and unfeeling toward the child.

In 1964, Bernard Rimland, a psychologist and parent of an autistic son, published *Infantile Autism: The Syndrome and its Implication for a Neural Theory of Behavior* in which he attacked the theory. But Bettelheim refused to consider an alternative theory and in 1967, he published *The Empty Fortress: Infantile Autism and the Birth of Self*, in which he compared autism to being a prisoner in a concentration camp.

Bettelheim published studies that reported an 80 percent success rate with treating children with autism in his school. In his studies, he chose the subjects and pronounced the positive outcomes by himself. His claims were not based on any real evidence, but simply his need to claim success for himself, and to protect his livelihood and the school. It is not surprising that professionals were unable to duplicate his studies, and achieve such a high success rate. It was finally revealed that Bettelheim had created false studies showing fantastic success rates, in order to bring money to his school.

Biological Psychiatry

The 20th century became a time of great belief in science and our ability to cure most anything. Some psychiatrists wanted to align themselves more closely with medicine, so new medical techniques were quickly adopted and tried. In 1938, psychiatrists started using barbiturate narcosis, insulin coma, and metrazol convulsion on mentally ill patients in the institutions with great excitement and promises of remissions and cures. Electroshock and lobotomy procedures soon followed. At the same time, desperate parents wanted to believe that medical doctors could cure mental illness.

Lobotomy (psychosurgery)

A lobotomy is a surgical procedure that destroys brain tissue in the prefrontal lobes. It was introduced to professionals by Egas Moniz (1877-1963). It wasn't based on science, but on the willingness of psychiatrists to believe in the words of a well-respected colleague that the procedure was beneficial.

The surgery was performed by drilling two holes in the top of the head, inserting a whisk-like instrument through the holes, and moving the instrument back and forth to destroy brain tissue. This was done without direct view of the brain, so it was impossible to determine how much tissue was destroyed, or the exact location. Therefore, the physician would sometimes repeat the procedure to destroy more brain tissue, if he felt the first operation had not been successful.

Walter Jackson Freeman, II, M.D. (1895-1972) and neurosurgeon James Winston Watts (1904-1994) introduced another method of lobotomy that was widely used in the United States. They inserted an instrument, such as an ice pick, hammered through the bone above the eye socket, and swished it around the brain tissue to destroy it.

Desperation makes parents vulnerable to someone in a position of authority telling us what to do. Even the educated and wealthy are vulnerable to cruel compassion promoted by professionals. President John F. Kennedy had a sister named Rose Marie "Rosie" Kennedy (1918-2005) who was mildly retarded (IQ 60-70 range). Her father, Joe Kennedy, was told that a new procedure called a lobotomy would help Rosie. In 1941, at the age of 23, Rosie was given a lobotomy at St. Elizabeth's Hospital and as a result, she would spend the rest of her life in an institution.

In December, 2013, Michael M. Phillips wrote an article in The Wall Street Journal, *"The Lobotomy Files/Family Scars: Torn by Choices made a Lifetime ago."* He wrote about some of the families of 2,000 veterans of World War II who were lobotomized by the VA and state hospitals. Mr. Phillips said that most people – including the VA – forgot about this history, but the families continue to be affected. Mr. Phillips described the guilt and regret of the family members, who allowed their loved ones to be lobotomized. The article noted one son died as a result of the lobotomy and all lost their independence.

Egas Moniz was given the Nobel Prize in Medicine in 1949 for his discovery of lobotomy. Lobotomy peaked in 1949 with over 5,000 operations. It is estimated that over 18,000 lobotomies were performed in the United States, before fading away in the 1950's, with the introduction of drugs for the treatment of mental problems.

Autism was classified as a form of schizophrenia until 1980 and this was justification for performing lobotomies on both children and adults. I am horrified that we easily forget how we mistreat our fellow man, including children. The families knew the procedure did not work, as it destroyed the person that they knew and yet, the medical profession continued to promote this surgical technique that destroyed brain tissue, while ignoring the devastation that it brought to the patients and families.

How could doctors continue to treat patients with lobotomy when there was so much evidence that it did not work? The Rockefeller Foundation provided huge funds to support the science-based treatments. Moniz said lobotomy was justified, based on experiments on chimps, designed to identify deficits in the frontal lobes, resulting from injury to the area. It was an unexpected observation from these experiments that the animals were calmer after the surgery. Moniz assumed humans would be calmer after lobotomy as well. All scientists receiving funds needed to claim positive results to ensure the funds would continue. When you want to see positive results, it becomes easy to do so.

There were other medical personnel who would benefit from the lobotomies. Neurosurgeons scrambled for patients in the 1930's and fees for lobotomies would quickly enrich their lifestyles. State governments were hopeful that lobotomies would send patients home and reduce the costs to the state. When one has so much to gain, it becomes difficult to see any negative outcomes to the surgery.

Electroshock Treatment

Electroshock (ECT) was first tried on dogs to determine where to apply the electrodes, as well as determine the proper dose to create convulsions, but avoid death. The medical experimenters were eager to try it on a human. In 1938, in Rome, a man was found wandering about the railway station, talking to himself and hallucinating. The police took him to the hospital for observation.

Dr. Ugo Cerletti (1877-1963), an Italian neurologist credited with the discovery of ECT therapy for use in psychiatry, led the experiments for the use of electroshock. This patient was taken into a room and Cerletti and colleagues gave the man three shocks with increasing dosages, with the third dose producing a full convulsion. When the patient woke up, he had no memory of what had happened. Dr. Cerletti gave the patient eleven shock treatments, then proclaimed the patient well and he returned home. The man's wife reported that the symptoms returned three months after returning home, but psychiatrists claimed the man was perfectly well a year after the treatments.

The use of electroshock treatments spread rapidly with great claims of success. Electroshock was used for depression, also called neurasthenia or nervous exhaustion. It was theorized that the treatment should stimulate the nervous system. What better way than shock therapy that created convulsions? Initially, the treatment often resulted in such violent convulsions that the patients would break bones. These side effects were ignored, since the focus was on curing the depression.

Psychiatrists decided to extend the experimental treatment to other mental conditions, such as schizophrenia. Since autism was considered a form of schizophrenia, the treatments included children. From 1940 to 1956, electroconvulsive treatment was used on more than 500 children at Bellevue Hospital in New York City. Dr. Lauretta Bender (1897-1987), a highly respected pediatric psychiatrist, administered electroshock experiments on more than 200 children, ages 3-12 years, at Bellevue Hospital from 1940-1953.

Publicly, Dr. Bender claimed that the results of the therapy were positive, but in private memos, she expressed frustration over mental health issues caused by her treatment. In 1954, a study of about fifty of Bender's patients found that nearly all were worse off after the therapy, and that some had become suicidal after the treatment.

Dr. Bender continued electroshock treatment with children at Creedmoor State Hospital Children's Services in New York from 1956-1969. Well-intentioned professionals can become quite zealous in their chosen treatment of our children and parents are quite vulnerable to someone in authority claiming they can cure autism.

One of Dr. Bender's patients was a child named Guy, who was diagnosed with autism. He was the son of Jacqueline Susanne, author of **Valley of the Dolls**. Dr. Bender convinced Susanne and her husband, that Guy could be successfully treated by electroshock treatment. Guy returned home from Bender's care a nearly lifeless child. Susanne later told people that Bender had *"destroyed"* her son. Guy was confined to institutions after his treatment.

In the 1960's, patient rights groups began protesting electroshock treatment and by 1983, thirty-three (33) state governments had passed regulations regarding ECT, with some states banning it altogether. Psychiatrists counterattacked by forming a task force and reporting positive results with ECT. The National Institute of Health held a conference and concluded that medical schools should restore ECT training.

In 1990, the American Psychiatric Association issued a report on the effectiveness of ECT for major depression, bipolar disorder and psychotic schizophrenia. It is interesting how easy it is to overlook any evidence against something one wants to believe in. Apparently the 1954 study of Dr. Bender's patients was ignored or forgotten. The controversy continues into the present, with some countries banning electroshock (electroconvulsive therapy), and some countries limiting its use on minors.

In the 1960's Laura Bender started using LSD on autistic children with the expectation that it would make them talk. She experimented on a total of eighty-nine children and published numerous articles. The experiments did not produce good science and by the end of the 1960's, LSD had become a popular recreational drug and the government restricted access, so it was difficult to obtain.

Psychiatric Medications Marketed to General Public

In the 1950's, drugs were being introduced that could be used to treat psychiatric disorders. Thorazine was a tranquilizer that was used for surgical patients. It would limit the patient's ability to move, but not put them to sleep. Some psychiatrists tried it to calm manic patients and it was not a cure, but it controlled behavior and made the patients more easily managed by staff.

There was a major side effect from the drug. Thorazine produces a progressive degeneration of movement, such as that seen in Parkinson's. The symptoms are called tardive dyskinesia and include a shuffling gait, loss of facial movements, and drooling, but these problems were easily ignored when the focus was on the benefits of managing behaviors of patients.

The drug makers realized that money could be made by marketing psychiatric drugs to the general public. The drug manufacturers extended the psychiatric diagnosis to everyone with the idea that a little pill could cure sadness, nervousness, and dealing with the stress of living. The public accepted the notion that everyone could have depression or nervousness that required drug treatment, and it became common for people to use tranquilizers (Valium, Librium), and antidepressants (Zoloft, Elavil, Prozac). It was no longer an embarrassment to have a mental illness or disability. Labels were extended to become a spectrum, where they could be applied to anyone.

When the drug therapies psychiatrists used for mental disorders soared in popularity with the general public, other physicians started prescribing these drugs. Since any physician could prescribe drugs, people could be treated on an outpatient basis with even a family physician. This resulted in psychiatry losing authority over patients with mental disabilities.

The medications prescribed most often for schizophrenia are antipsychotics. They are meant to ease the effects of hallucinations and delusions. I am concerned we are too quick to accept antipsychotics for our children with disabilities, in an attempt to restrain them, rather than understanding behaviors as a reflection of brain differences. This is not a cure and can have devastating side effects. It hasn't been that long ago that psychiatry thought of autism as a form of schizophrenia.

Changing and Elusive Labels

After WWII, psychiatrists working with veterans needed a diagnostic manual that would give credibility to a diagnosis that would enable victims of war to receive services. The American Psychiatric Association started a standardized psychiatric classification system, resulting in the 1952 publication of the Diagnostic and Statistical Manual of Mental Disorders (DSM-I).

By the time DSM III was being prepared for 1980 publication, there were major changes in the labels. After 1971, Vietnam Veterans pressured psychiatrists to add *"Post Traumatic Stress Disorder (PTSD)."* Epilepsy and homosexuality were eliminated from the manual, because they were no longer considered a *"mental illness."* Changing attitudes made abuse of alcohol and drugs a *"disease,"* rather than a character flaw, and made the condition eligible for research and funding. Autism was considered a form of schizophrenia until 1980 when the DSM III changed it to a *"pervasive developmental disability,"* reflecting the new political label for federal legislation, increasing funds for research and education.

"Disability" is a legal term used in the federal laws such as the Individuals with Disabilities Education Act (IDEA) and Section 504 of the Rehabilitation Act. "Disorder" is a medical term from the Diagnostic and Statistical Manual of Mental Disorders of the American Psychiatric Association.

Autism was a label that was associated with a poor prognosis or outcome and this view was not going to make it acceptable for research and educational funds. In preparation for the next publication – the DSM IV – professionals with a different vision of autism, such as Lorna Wing a British psychiatrist, heavily influenced the changes in diagnosis. She pushed for the addition of Asperger's Syndrome, people who are described as socially odd, but not mentally retarded. She also wanted the restrictive nomenclature of autism to be expanded to include more children. This would increase the popularity of the diagnosis, for it would demonstrate a better prognosis and increase the number of people with the label. This increase in the number of people with the diagnosis served to justify more funding for the condition.

In 2015, Steve Silberman published his New York Times bestseller, **Neurotribes, The Legacy of Autism and the Future of Neurodiversity.** The book gives society a view of autism as those who are geniuses, who can contribute to the technology industry, be self-advocates, and policymakers. The media loves this approach and there are television shows and movies portraying autism in this manner. Those with Asperger's Syndrome do not want to be associated with those on the rest of the spectrum and I certainly appreciate that. I acknowledge that most people do not want to face the reality of severe autism. My concern is the book gives a skewed idealized representation of those with autism and their needs, because it focuses on the high end and essentially ignores the rest of the spectrum.

Dr. Allen Frances, Chair of the DSM-IV task force, published *Saving Normal: An Insider's Revolt against Out-of-Control Psychiatric Diagnosis, DSM-5, Big Pharma, and the Medicalization of Ordinary Life* where he stated that classic autism is severe and easy to recognize and the line between Asperger's and normality is blurred. Dr. Frances also noted that the changes in the diagnostic criteria in DSM-IV resulted in too many children being diagnosed with attention deficit, autism, and childhood bipolar disorder. The diagnosis of autism has gone from four to five children in ten thousand, to one in eighty.

Television began to portray autism as an individual who is a quirky genius with endearing repetitive behaviors, such as Sheldon on "The Big Bang Theory." I have encountered teachers who refer to individuals with autism as "all so smart." I recently found a book (2002) by Norm Ledgin called *Asperger's and Self-Esteem: Insight and Hope through famous role models.* Some of the role models – such as Einstein, Mozart, Darwin, and Jefferson – all supposedly had Asperger's. How difficult can it be to accept a diagnosis of Autism Spectrum Disorder when it is associated with great minds from the past?

After David was diagnosed in 1988 with autistic disorder, I visited schools to find a place for David. Much to my surprise, there were schools isolated where one would never know they existed. Although there was some push toward inclusion of disabled children in regular classrooms, this was strongly resisted. I observed separate wings of the schools designated for disabled children and I saw buses transport disabled children to the back of the school, as opposed to where the other buses dropped off children. I saw a school next to a regular school, but separated by a fence. This was defined as "inclusion" by the school authorities.

We need to remember that attitudes in society change slowly. We have an aversion to confronting the disturbing reality of severe autism and disabled children. We institutionalized these people to keep them out of sight of society. With the addition of children with Asperger's to the spectrum, society views only the top of the spectrum, as if the reality of severe autism does not exist.

There has been considerable criticism (even from psychiatrists) against the most recent publication of the American Psychiatric Association, DSM-5, in 2013. In Gary Greenberg's book titled, *The Book of Woe: The DSM and the Unmaking of Psychiatry*, published in the same year, makes an interesting read about the problems in the field.

The DSM-5 combined all the different types of pervasive developmental disabilities under one label called *"Autism Spectrum Disorder (ASD)"*. One reason for this change was the inability of diagnosticians to agree on patient diagnoses. The label given to an individual depended on the diagnostician and was not applied consistently.

The manual of the DSM lists preposterous disorders as behaviors with no physical cause to support a diagnosis. Medical diagnoses should give one an idea of treatment and prognosis, but the psychiatric diagnosis fails to do this. I agree with Dr. Frances who suggests that the American Psychiatric Association should no longer have total control over the nomenclature. Brain science now can explain autism and give us new teaching and parenting methods.

Psychiatry and Neurology

Have you ever wondered why psychiatry defines autism and not neurology? If autism is a brain deficit – a neurological problem – then why isn't it defined as such? I was surprised to find the answer in history – back in the 1800's.

In 1844, superintendents (psychiatrists) of thirteen mental institutions formed the Association of Medical Superintendents of American Institutions for the Insane (AMSAII). The members of this organization were mainly concerned with the administration of the institutions.

By the end of the civil war (1864), the United States was experiencing a variety of changes. There was competition for the development of different specialties and disagreement over how to handle the problems in society. Neurology became a rising profession from the clinical experience treating neurologically injured soldiers in the civil war. They felt they were involved in the new "scientific" developments in medicine; and, therefore, they should be the experts treating the mentally disabled.

In 1875, eighteen physicians established the American Neurological Association (ANA). The neurologists prohibited psychiatrists from joining the newly formed ANA, claiming they were more qualified to treat mental illness than the psychiatrists who managed institutions. The asylums or mental institutions were isolated from hospitals where medical doctors treated the ill, so this created more division between psychiatry and other medical specialties. They were attempting to take control of psychiatry by claiming psychiatrists were not "scientific" and they were "merely managers of institutions". The next year, neurologists established the Journal of Nervous and Mental Diseases to promote neurology as science-based. Therefore, considerable conflict existed between psychiatry and neurology.

American neurologist, George Miller Beard (1839-1883), created a neurological niche that reduced the antagonism between neurology and psychiatry. Dr. Beard facilitated the acceptance of neurasthenia or nervous exhaustion (later known as depression), as a functional disorder that was curable, using a mild electrical massage to stimulate the nervous system. This explanation had wide appeal to people needing to believe it was a cure for a disorder, rather than a chronic untreatable mental illness. The theory suggested that people suffering from neurasthenia were more likely higher class and highly successful.

Associating neurology with ideas from science, such as the electrical transmission of nerve impulses, gave it more value and acceptance. The argument followed that psychiatry was not "science based." By the end of the nineteenth century, neurologists had successfully established themselves as experts of neurasthenia based on science and created a community treatment program by blurring the line between normality and abnormality. Their funding source was directly from their patients, as they recruited from the higher income levels. Once this professional base was established, they no longer needed to attack psychiatrists.

Psychiatry maintained the authority to label mental disorders, but those labels continue to ignore neurology. The American Psychiatric Association has come under considerable criticism over its nomenclature. In 2004, V.S. Ramachandran in **A Brief Tour of Human Consciou5ness** (the 5 is not a typo) wrote that *"it is only a matter of time before psychiatry becomes just another branch of neurology."* It appears that the battle may not be over.

Eric Kandal writes in **The Disordered Mind: What Unusual Brains Tell Us about Ourselves (2018),** a prediction that *"neurology and psychiatry will merge into a common clinical discipline that focuses increasingly on the patient as an individual with particular genetic predispositions to health and disease."*

History reveals that our attitudes toward disabilities influence our treatment of children with autism. In the 20th Century, we had many professionals who did great harm to people with disabilities in the name of science, using electroshock and lobotomy. Some professionals – such as Bettelheim – blamed parents for causing the disability, to silence them from objecting to their children being taken away to institutions.

Psychiatric labels are constantly changing and influenced more by politics and society than science. Autism was initially excluded from the legal definition "developmentally disabled" because it was considered a mental illness (schizophrenia), so autism did not receive the funding for research and education. Psychiatrists changed the label of autism from a mental illness to a developmental disability and changed the diagnostic criteria to include children who were socially odd, but did not test as mentally retarded.

The DSM-IV added Asperger's Syndrome, a category for children with social oddities but better language and no mental retardation. In addition, they expanded the diagnostic criteria for Autistic Disorder, resulting in more children being diagnosed as "autistic."

In 2013 many labels became spectrums, where they could be applied to anyone. The DSM- 5 consolidated all the pervasive developmental disabilities into a spectrum – Autism Spectrum Disorder (provided in back of book). Apparently, it became necessary to combine the various labels, because clinicians could not agree on a diagnosis for an individual, and the label was determined more by the clinician than science.

The "Aspies" did not like being associated with others on the autism spectrum. They promoted the idea that they are geniuses, who contribute to the technology industry, are self-advocates, and policymakers. Books, television and movies pushed a social vision of autism as people with sensory and social challenges, but who can live independently and are highly intelligent. This view has started to dominant society, so those on the rest of the spectrum have been ignored or forgotten.

The DSM -5 also eliminated the diagnostic criteria for Asperger's syndrome from DSM-IV that stated *"there is no delay in development of age-appropriate self-help skills and adaptive behavior."* This was because the great hope for improved outcomes with those with Asperger's syndrome did not occur. In 2007, White and colleagues published in the <u>Journal of Autism and Developmental Disorders</u> stating, *"Placement in regular education may inadvertently widen the gap in higher functioning children if the teaching focus on traditional academics overshadows teaching other social and self-care skills these children need."* This is in sharp contrast to the prevailing societal perspective.

The core features in the DSM 5 are social interaction/communication deficits and restrictive, repetitive behaviors. The medical diagnosis does not include the lack of observation and imitation, lack of generalization and strengths and deficits in sensory processing. Behaviors are labeled, but not understood. Dr. Francis, Chair of the DSM-IV task force, writes that the medical diagnosis was meant for clinical purposes and not research or educational purposes, although that is precisely what it is used for.

If we create treatments for children with autism based on unreliable diagnostic information, then the treatments will be inappropriate. We must acknowledge our mistakes, so we do not repeat them. The psychiatric label includes too diverse a group and the focus has turned to the higher functioning without mental retardation and ignores the rest of the spectrum. This review indicates that the psychiatric label of autism does not properly fit into the puzzle, because it does not describe the neurological impairments. It is time to define the symptoms of autism based on brain structure and function. This is discussed in **Section Two – The Brain and Autism.**

Chapter 4

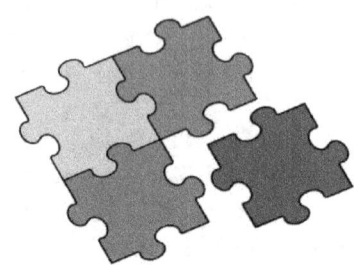

Applied Behavior Analysis (ABA)

"No Matter how big the lie is, just repeat it often enough and the masses will regard it as the truth."   John F. Kennedy

Applied Behavior Analysis (ABA) Programs are touted as beneficial for children with autism. ABA therapy programs are based on the Ivar Lovaas UCLA experiment in 1970 in which he applied behavioral treatment to young children with autism. UCLA is one of the funded lab schools established by the government. In 1987, Dr. Lovaas published a paper in the Journal of Consulting and Clinical Psychology titled, *"Behavioral Treatment and Normal Educational and Intellectual Functioning in Young Autistic Children."* This is the study that is frequently cited (but seldom read) as the scientific basis of ABA.

History of Behaviorism

Before reviewing this study, a brief history of the development and theory behind ABA is needed. Behaviorism evolved from experimental psychology that began in the 1800's in Europe to try to understand the processes of the mind. Wilhelm Wundt (1832-1920) established the first psychology laboratory in Leipzig, Germany and he trained many psychologists, who would later establish psychology laboratories throughout Europe and the United States. Wundt studied reaction times (how long it took a person to complete a task, such as a math problem) and he developed the method of introspection, asking people to describe their thoughts, when he presented a series of objects.

John B. Watson (1878-1958) disagreed with psychology's focus on mental processes and he developed the field of behaviorism that seemed more scientific, because it focused only on observed behaviors. He believed that all animals (including humans) learned from the environment (triggers or stimuli) and by understanding the stimuli, one could predict the responses. He believed infants were born knowing nothing (blank slates) and acquired all knowledge through the environment.

Behaviorists believe that all behaviors can be predicted and controlled and all students can learn the same information given an appropriate environment. The theory was initially called "behavior modification." The theory emphasizes rewards and punishments in changing behaviors. The desire to learn is assumed to be driven by the stimulus-response relationship, and it assumes the child can understand what is being taught.

Burrhus Frederic (B.F.) Skinner (1904-1990) and Ole Ivar Lovaas (1927-2010) were two psychologists who promoted and extended the theory of behaviorism. Skinner developed the theory of behaviorism with his work on rats and pigeons and then applied these ideas to humans. He wrote a fictional account of his views of the utopian society in the 1948 novel, **Walden Two**, where all of society's problems are solved by behaviorism. He also wrote **Verbal Behavior** in 1957 where he applied behavioral theory to language acquisition.

Behaviorism became widely accepted in the 1960's and was based on the idea of the blank slate and all learning occurred from outside input. As discussed in Chapter 2 _The Pendulum Swings_, the genetic determinism of the late 19th and early 20th century swung the opposite way to the idea that everything is determined by the environment and not genetics. Behaviorism became outdated in the 1990's when brain science provided evidence of the fallacy of the theory.

Behaviorism and the Treatment of Autism

Behaviorism is based on the theory of operant or instrumental conditioning. Our behaviors are instrumental in that they are a means to an end, or done for a purpose. We buy food for the purpose of eating. Skinner chose the term "operant" to describe the idea that animals operate on their environments to produce effects. Operant conditioning is the learning process in which an action's consequences determine the likelihood that the action will be performed in the future. This is the belief that behaviors that are positively reinforced (praised, rewarded) will increase; and behaviors that are negatively reinforced (punished, ignored) will extinguish.

Parents understand the theory – if not the psychobabble – that if a child runs out into the street, a spanking or grabbing the child with a loud "*No*" will likely prevent the child from running into the street in the future. Parents praise and reward behavior that they want the child to continue, such as getting good grades or doing their chores.

Behaviorists blamed parents for giving the wrong kinds and patterns of reinforcement resulting in aberrant behaviors of autism. Therefore, the child was removed from the home and placed in an institution. Ivar Lovaas, Ph.D. began behavioral treatment experiments in the 1960's using children with autism from a local institution. Lovaas became infamous for his use of punishment on children with autism. He used a "Hot-Shot", which was a cattle prod, to deliver electric shocks to eliminate aberrant behaviors. There was great controversy over the use of punishment, therefore Lovaas used the term "aversives."

A commercial product was developed called the "Self-Injurious Behavior Inhibiting System (SIBI)." It was a helmet worn by the child and a parent or practitioner could deliver a remote-controlled shock, whenever the child showed unwanted behaviors. This use of punishment on children with autism created great controversy. Some groups – such as the Autism Society of America – took a strong position against the use of punishments. Although Lovaas toned down his use of punishment, his prior use of the Hot-Shot (cattle prod) made it difficult for him to obtain support from parents and other professionals for his behavior modification.

Lovaas learned that after working with the children from the institution, they quickly regressed, so his next experiment used young children with autism living at home. He published **Teaching Developmentally Disabled Children: The ME Book** in 1981 that contained an explicit set of programs to help parents and teachers. In the preface of the book, he wrote that in the beginning, he made the mistake of assuming only professionals could provide treatment, and he isolated parents from the program. He changed his approach with the child's treatment being provided by parents and teachers in the child's home and school. The professionals trained the parents and teachers, and then provided consultation.

Current ABA programs claim only highly trained specialists can provide therapy for children with autism, and this is a deviation from Lovaas, who came to the belief that parents were capable of being therapists. The Lovaas approach is called "Applied Behavior Analysis (ABA)," as this sounds more professional than behavior modification. ABA has been highly touted as a beneficial treatment for children with autism. A close review of his 1987 study will help us determine if it is a valid and scientific study that can provide benefits to children with autism.

The Lovaas Experiment

Lovaas correctly noted that normal children learn from their environments (observation and imitation), but autistic children do not learn from their environments. Therefore, he hypothesized that *"construction of a special, intense and comprehensive learning environment for very young autistic children would allow some of them to catch up with their normal peers by first grade."* His hypothesis clearly states his expectation that his learning program would have a positive result. He had strong personal motivation to promote his program as beneficial for children with autism, and proceeded to design an experiment to prove his belief.

The Lovaas report indicates that subjects selected for this experiment had to meet three criteria: 1) Independent diagnosis of autism; 2) Chronological age of less than 40 months, if mute, and less than 46 months, if echolalic (repeating something heard either immediately or delayed); and 3) Prorated Mental Age of 11 months or more at a chronological age of 30 months. According to Lovaas, this requirement for a mental age of 11 months eliminated 15% of the referrals.

Three Groups

Experimental Group. There were originally 21 students in the experimental group. Two dropped out within six months, but no explanation was given, as to why they left the program. The 19 students of this group were each assigned several well-trained student therapists who worked (each part-time) with the student, for an average of 40 hours per week, for 2 or more years. Parents were trained to be part of the treatment team, so treatment could take place for almost all of the subjects' waking hours, 365 days a year. There were 16 boys and 3 girls in this group. The average chronological age in this group was 35 months, so they are younger than the Control Group 1. Lovaas reported that 10 of the 19 children in the experimental group were referred for neurological examinations, but he failed to identify if they were among the nine students that he claimed recovered.

Control Group 1. There were 19 students in this group and they received less than 10 hours of one-to-one treatment per week. They also attended small special education classes within their community. The students in this control group were 6 months older (average chronological age 41 months) and contained more girls (11 boys and 8 girls). Since autism is more prevalent in boys (4:1), and a higher proportion of autistic girls have mental retardation, this indicates that the two groups could not be considered equal for comparison. Nothing was said about parent training, so one wonders if this is the important variable related to outcome.

In this control group, 15 of the 19 were referred to a neurologist, with 1 showing signs of neurological damage. One would assume, that a referral for a neurological examination, indicated more questionable observable behaviors, perhaps more severe. This would also indicate that the control group had a larger contingency of more severely involved children (as well as more girls) and was not an appropriate control group.

Control Group 2. This group consisted of 21 students selected from a larger group of 62 that were studied by B.J. Freeman. The students for this group were selected, if they were 42 months old or younger when first tested, had IQ scores above 40 at intake, and had follow-up testing at 6 years of age. These students were treated like those in Control Group 1, but were not treated by the UCLA Lovaas group.

Treatment for Experimental Group

First Year. Treatment goals were directed toward reducing aberrant behaviors, teaching response to verbal requests, imitation, appropriate toy play, and *"promoting extension of the treatment into the family."*

Second Year. Treatment goals were directed toward expressive language, early abstract language and interaction with peers. Treatment was also extended into a regular preschool. Students were required to go to preschools where the teacher helped carry out the treatment program.

Third Year. Treatment goals were directed toward expressing emotions and pre-academic tasks (reading, writing, and arithmetic). After preschool, placement was determined by the public school. Those students who attended a regular kindergarten received only 10 hours of ABA per week – down from 40 hours per week during the first two years. All students who successfully completed a regular kindergarten, also completed regular first grade.

Results

Lovaas stated that 9 of the 19 children in the experimental group "recovered," because their IQ scores were within the normal range and they were able to attend regular first grade. He attributed his ABA program as the cause of their recovery. Yet, science does not prove cause and effect – it only demonstrates a high correlation between a variable and an outcome. Lovaas noted that the improved IQ scores were consistent with Dr. Leo Kanner's theory that autistic children potentially possess normal intelligence. In other words, Lovaas believed mental retardation can be cured – a common belief (or wishful thinking) from the 1970's, as discussed in chapter two.

Lovaas reported the nine (9) successful students all responded to verbal imitations within the first three months. Verbal imitation is the first step to teaching the child to talk. It involves imitation of sounds and words. He also noted that the ten (10) remaining students from the experimental group all failed to learn verbal imitation, but were more adept at matching visual stimuli, so they were more visual learners. Lovaas suggested that if the child does not imitate sounds within two or three months, then the parent should consider minimizing or dropping the program.

In addition to only 9 children responding to verbal imitation, there were other variables in the experiment that may have been significant. The experimental group included punishment to extinguish unwanted behaviors, but the control group did not include punishment. Lovaas felt that the study could not be replicated, or achieve good outcomes, without the use of punishment.

The experimental group included training of parents and preschool teachers, who also provided therapy. It would be interesting to know if the 9 successful students received more therapy from parents than the rest of the group. Another variable was the experimental group all attended regular preschools but the control group attended special education classes. Was this the variable that was important to the outcome?

Lovaas stated the prorated mental age was the only variable pretested that was significantly related to outcome. It is well recognized in the professional literature that autistic children who start with higher IQ's and more verbal ability are more successful in school. The Lovaas experiment seems to confirm this, as the successful students had higher prorated mental age and responded to verbal imitation within three months of beginning therapy. If this is the case, then the "recovery" of the nine successful students was more related to their innate brain function and not related to "therapy."

The successful students from the Lovaas study should be compared closely to other children with autism, who have become successful without ABA. We already reviewed three positive outcomes from the 11 children identified by Kanner. They did not receive ABA therapy. In addition, one student in the Control Group II headed by B.J. Freeman achieved a normal IQ (99) and placement in a regular first grade. It would be interesting to compare this child's treatment to the treatment of the children in the Lovaas experimental group and to the three positive outcomes from the Kanner group as none of them received ABA. In other words, I contend there will be a few children diagnosed as autistic, but who are not retarded, and will be more successful regardless of the therapy.

Outcome Measures

Good science tries to control the variables. Since outcomes were based on IQ scores, that is the variable being tested. Lovaas apparently thought he was uncovering the hidden intelligence in autistic children by claiming some of the students were "recovered." This is a continuation of the idea that mental retardation can be cured (discussed in Chapter 2 _The Pendulum Swings_) and this is not true.

A variable can only be tested properly if two groups are equal to start with (start with same IQ levels). Yet, Lovaas reported that the experimental group was younger at the start of the program, and they started with a higher prorated mental age, greater toy play, and fewer aberrant behaviors. Therefore, the two groups were not comparable, so any results have no validity. The Lovaas experiment lacks scientific credibility and used mental testing to make it appear "scientific."

IQ scores are the most common outcome measures in research and this is inappropriate for several reasons. First, IQ scores can change based on the examiner, how the child feels that day, and with each administration of the test. In research, the same examiner should administer the test in the beginning and the end of the experiment, without knowledge of which group the child belongs (control or experimental). If different tests are used at the end of an experiment, then any conclusions may be unreliable.

Secondly, IQ only predicts how well one can do in school and it does not measure practical skills (life skills). Thirdly, an IQ test is not a measure of whether the treatment produces generalization of skills to other situations or improvement in practical skills for children with autism, leading to increased independence and self-reliance. Yet, researchers continue to rely on a number on a test, because it seems more "scientific."

Dr. Richard J. Hair, professor of pediatric neurology at the University of California, Irvine and researcher at the MIND Institute in Albuquerque, NM, published an article in 2014 in Frontiers in Systems Neuroscience called *Increased Intelligence is a Myth (so far)*. He writes that you cannot use intelligence tests to demonstrate the effectiveness of an intervention and he suggests that a new type of measurement is required based on the brain.

Dr. Hair also noted that IQ scores are not a unit of measurement - such as length or weight. Units of measurement are ratio scales and IQ scores are interval scales. In other words, IQ scores are not easily interpreted. The author writes there is no scientific evidence for any claims that increased intelligence results from any treatment, including early childhood education.

When the therapy results in an improvement in IQ scores, we assume one caused the other. In reality all that has happened is two events occurred in succession. Magical thinking occurs when we connect two successive events and conclude that the first event caused the second. IQ scores in young children are not stable, and scores should improve as children become more verbal, since the test measures knowledge gained, and relies on verbal ability. In addition, IQ scores can vary from one test session to another, based on the experience of the person administering the test, how the child feels that day, and if it is a different test from the one given previously.

The second outcome measure used by Lovaas was placement in a regular classroom, as this assumes the child can function more normally. I agree with the National Research Council (2001) that writes, *"The usefulness of placement in the regular education classes as an outcome measure is limited, because placement may be related to the many variables other than the characteristics of the child (e.g., prevailing trends in inclusion, availability of other services)."*

Building an ABA Industry

Lovaas was disappointed in the lack of support for his treatment method. He noted colleagues interested in other areas of investigation discounted his work, and two professionals (unnamed), with the Autism Society of America, called his work a fraud. Lovaas felt he was not being appreciated and he could not accept any criticism of his methods.

Lovaas was a friend of Bernie Rimland (1928-2006), a psychologist, who had helped establish the Autism Society of America. Rimland was outspokenly supportive of the punishment program that used the Hot-Shot cattle prod, even though the Autism Society took a position opposed to it. In 1987, Rimland hired an ABA trainer from the Lovaas program to work with his son, Mark, who has autism. It wasn't long before Lovaas teamed up with Bernie Rimland to promote the method to parents.

Rimland convinced Lovaas to sell his program to parents, and Rimland was in the perfect position to help him accomplish that, because he had been involved with starting the Autism Society of America. Rather than trying to convert professional colleagues to support his method, Lovaas and Rimland worked together to help parents teach their children using ABA methods.

Professionals can often become overzealous when they present their research findings. Lovaas used the word "recovered" and to many parents, this translated as "cured." In 1993 when Catherine Maurice published her book ***Let Me Hear Your Voice: A Family's Triumph over Autism*** (that included a preface by Bernie Rimland and an afterward from Ivar Lovaas), how could any parent not seek ABA treatment for a child that was being so strongly promoted as a "cure"?

When professionals realized what was happening, they jumped at the opportunity to create a specialty that would provide ABA treatments to families, and a livelihood for properly trained ABA specialists. This is not based on the Lovaas' theory, because he felt parents should be trained to work with their children. Despite the fact many professionals did not initially support ABA, once it became popular with parents, ABA programs increased, although some ignored the lessons from Lovaas and only incorporated aspects of the theory that were convenient for them.

Applied Behavior Analysis (ABA) has become an extensive commercial venture that is based on the Lovaas claim that his program enabled nine children to "recover" from autism. ABA has also become known as Discrete Trial (DT) and Intensive Behavior Intervention (IBI). The ABA programs are very expensive and time consuming, but that doesn't stop parents from trying anything that might help their children. Parents have gone to court to require school systems to pay for this teaching approach. We often hear that the only effective treatment is ABA.

In the summer of 2016, the Autism Society of N.C. published an article offering lifelong ABA intervention services that can only be delivered under the supervision of a licensed psychologist. The article stated that the actual delivery of the services must be provided by someone with extensive training and certification. The interventions can be from 10 to 40 hours per week with the claim that more hours are more beneficial. Isn't it interesting that the Lovaas program developed for young children has been extended to all ages? In addition, the program has been changed from training parents and teachers to the use of only highly trained professionals being able to provide treatment.

A recent article in the News & Observer, Raleigh, N.C. **"New Mandate for Autism Care Lifts Financial Strain"** discussed a new state law which will require all state-regulated insurance plans to cover Applied Behavior Analysis. The article noted that ABA treatment can cost up to $60,000 per year.

The extreme costs for educating children with autism can result in a backlash from the public paying for this treatment. In June 2014, Karen

Kaplan wrote an article in the <u>Los Angeles Times</u> called ***Autism's Cost Pegged at $236 Billion*** where she writes *"The amount spent annually on the disorder may be greater than the interest on the national debt. To put it into perspective, $1.43 million is more than enough to put five students through Harvard without any scholarships, grants or other discounts."* When the costs are seen as taking away from the education of typical children, we could see an attitude shift in society that is not as supportive toward people with disabilities. Parents of disabled children need to be more cautious of making demands for "therapy" because some self-serving professional tells you it is beneficial.

ABA was developed for young children with claims for recovery, but now it is offered as lifetime therapy indicating children with autism don't recover. ABA programs are shameless cons perpetrated on desperate parents and disabled children. The Big Lie is to tell parents that it is effective and repeating it so much that it has become regarded as truth.

Selling false hopes to desperate parents has got to be one of the lowest forms of human behavior. Speculation is not science. Selling ABA therapy to parents is pure propaganda. Behaviorists are trumpeting ABA as beneficial for students with autism. They have lobbied the federal government and managed to include ABA into the special education laws. As larger segments of the country have adopted the attitude that ABA is the only effective "treatment" for autism, it is not about science, but promoting self-interests for financial and professional benefits.

Flaws with Behaviorism (ABA)

Applied Behavior Analysis involves breaking a skill into steps and teaching the skill over and over. This aspect of ABA can be helpful to teach life skills, because it can teach to autistic strengths of attention to details and rote learning. But ABA theory has gone awry for numerous reasons: 1) It focuses on behaviors and ignores brain science; 2) It fails to recognize that not all behaviors can be taught; 3) It fails to teach meaningful skills; 4) It fails to teach skills in the various community environments where it is used; 5) It fails to give parents and teachers the skills to help children with autism and promotes the belief that only trained professionals can provide services at great expense to families.

Polly Yarnall, autism educational consultant, writes that ABA *"emphasizes compliance training, prompt dependence; heavy focus on behavioral approach may ignore underlying neurological aspects of autism, including issues of executive function and attention switching; may overstress child and/or family..."* The goals of ABA are to *"teach child how to learn by focusing on developing skills in attending, imitation, receptive/expressive language, pre-academics, and self-help."*

As noted earlier, behaviorism was established to focus only on observed behaviors and it ignored any possible causes of behavior. The theory assumes the child understands what is being taught, so the approach fails to teach meaningful skills from the child's perspective. It focuses on behavior as willful, rather than the result of a brain condition.

Some behaviors may be due to side effects of drugs. Darby Penney and Peter Stastny wrote about people in a state hospital in **The Lives They Left Behind.** They wrote about a seventy-eight year old woman who was given "behavior modification therapy" to alleviate strange movements and facial grimaces. This was noted to be inappropriate since the cause of the behaviors were from side effects of a drug treatment. In the 1950's, new drug treatments were introduced, including a drug called Thorazine, a tranquilizer or sedative. Thorazine causes side effects, such as shuffling gait, loss of facial movements and drooling. No amount of behavioral therapy was going to change these behaviors.

Behavior theory states that any behavior can be changed with ABA, but this is not true, as not all behaviors can be taught. Some behaviors are the result of how the brain functions and we do not know how to correct brain deficits. Dr. Restak, a neurologist, states in **The Modular Brain** (1994) science demonstrates brain function *"cannot be explained on the basis of a stimulus followed by a response."* Yet, professionals continue to promote the outdated theory to parents as beneficial for children with autism.

Secrets Revealed

Beneficial information from the study has been ignored or forgotten. Lovaas was intent on using the program with only very young children, so the current trend of lifetime therapy seems inappropriate. In addition, Lovaas reported that the 9 children who benefited from the program responded to speech imitation (auditory) within three months and the rest of the children (10) were more adept at matching visual stimuli, so they were visual learners and did not "recover." This indicates how children with autism will have different sensory strengths, and we must teach to the individual strengths and support the weak sensory processing. This is essential information that helps determine who might benefit from this behavioral strategy.

Dr. Lovaas felt aversives (punishment) were essential to the positive outcome in his study. He is known for his use of the Hot Shot cattle prod, but when he encountered condemnation for this behavior, he backed off. I don't believe we should physically punish children in order for them to learn. Behaviors are the result of differences in brain structure and function and sensory processing abilities, so learning by physical punishment is unnecessary.

ABA targets observed behaviors and teaches to the deficits. The National Research Council (2001) state *"In a behavioral approach, a child's behavioral repertoire is evaluated according to the presence of behavioral excesses – presence of abnormal behaviors or of an abnormal frequency of certain behaviors – and behavioral deficits – absence or low frequency of typical skills (Lovaas, 1987). Behavioral teaching strategies are then designed to increase a child's performance of deficit skills and decrease the behavioral excesses. These strategies involve identifying the target of teaching, determining the appropriate antecedent and consequence for the target behavior, and using systematic instruction and assessment to teach the target behavior and assess student progress."*

Unfortunately, researchers are developing teaching strategies that target a neurological deficit that cannot be changed, but must be accommodated. This is another example of professionals playing in their own sandbox and ignoring any other perspective on autism, or any evidence that science has advanced beyond this approach. When an approach is deemed effective, it is very difficult to get its followers to consider anything else. I discussed this in Chapter 2 with psychologists and IQ, and Chapter 3 with psychiatrists and lobotomy and electroshock.

Applied Behavior Analysis is just one teaching strategy used for children with autism, although it continues to be the main approach. There have been no studies to compare ABA to other teaching strategies, so it lacks scientific evidence. Brain science can now explain the behaviors in autism and this invalidates the theory of ABA.

The next chapter examines the history of educational research and factors influencing the research areas and goals.

Chapter 5

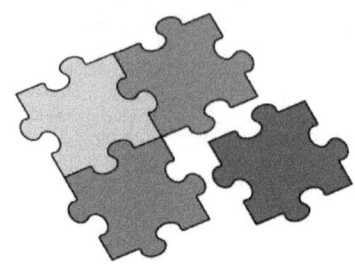

Educational Research
"The only source of knowledge is experience." Albert Einstein

In the 1960's, the Kennedy administration started funding University-based research centers or lab schools to search for the causes of mental retardation and the scientific treatments of the condition (including behavior modification or ABA). This shifted research from the state institutions to university lab centers, although state institutions initially provided the subjects for research.

In 2001, the National Research Council (NRC), with a grant from the Department of Education, reviewed ten of these University-based centers. One of these centers is the University of California at Los Angeles (UCLA) where Dr. Ivar Lovaas developed the Applied Behavior Analysis program that was discussed in the last chapter.

Most of the research centers are still based on an outdated theory of behaviorism that began in the 1960's. This means they believe anything and everything can be taught through stimulus-response learning. Behaviors are labeled as appropriate or deviant and teaching targets the deviant behaviors. There is no understanding of how different brain functions result in observed behaviors.

Research Guided by Politics

In the 1960's, the media and politicians touted the brutality of state institutions that segregated children with disabilities and deprived them of their civil rights. In 1975, the federal government passed law 94-142 IDEA (Individuals with Disabilities Education Act) requiring education for children with disabilities. At first disabled children were placed in special schools or special classes, but some parents were not satisfied with this type of education, because they wanted their disabled children in classes with nondisabled peers.

Parents based their argument on the idea of normalization – that disabilities were caused by institutions and lack of education and they simply needed opportunities to be in the environment with typical children learning "age-appropriate activities", and learning social skills from their nondisabled peers. This resulted in court cases supporting the education of children with disabilities in regular classrooms, including placing the burden on the school district to prove that a student cannot be educated successfully in the regular classroom (Oberti v. Board of Education, 1993).

The U.S. Supreme Court has stated that the Individuals with Disabilities Education Act (IDEA) require the education of disabled children with non-disabled children whenever possible (Board of Education v. Rowley 1982). There is a *"presumption that, among the alternative programs of education and training required by statute to be available, placement in a regular public school class is preferable to placement in a special public school class."*

Congress has promoted the importance of education of special education students in regular classes by requiring individual educational plans (IEP's) to include a statement describing how the child's disability affects her involvement and progress in the general curriculum and a statement of annual goals, including short-term objectives that are related to enabling the student to be involved and progress in the general curriculum (34 C.F.R. Secs. 300.320(a)(1) & (2).

The educational goals for disabled children should be based on the needs of the child and not directed by federal law. In **The Mind's Past** (1998), Michael Gazzaniga writes that when scientists try to satisfy the political system, it often results in skewing the results toward that goal.

The 37th Annual Report to Congress from the U.S. Department of Education on the Implementation of the Individuals with Disabilities Education Act, 2015, reported that inclusion was on the rise in the nation's schools. The data from this report stated *"95% of students age 6- 21 served under IDEA, Part B, were educated at least part of the day in regular classes. The remaining five percent of other special education students were served in other environments that consisted of separate schools, residential facilities, homebound/hospital environment, correctional facilities and parentally placed in private schools."*

In addition, from 2004 through 2013, the report noted a significant increase in inclusion in regular classes for 80% or more of the day from 51.8 percent to 62.1 percent, while the percentage of students attending regular classes 40% to 79% of the day dropped from 26.4% to 19.2%. Clearly, public schools are attempting to educate more children in regular classes to comply with the federal law.

With the long-term goal of disabled children attending a regular classroom, the short-term goals are specifically designed to enable teachers to handle disabled children in the classroom. The National Research Council (2001) stated goals for children with disabilities should include skills that enable the child to function independently in a regular classroom, such as *"responding to adult directions, independently participating in the routines of the classroom, expressing needs to adults (e.g., need to go to the bathroom), and requesting assistance of the adult."*

Although an educational plan is supposed to be individualized and developed based on the needs of the child, the goals are being changed based on the needs of the teacher trying to work with groups of children that include disabled children, and meet the requirements of federal laws. These goals distract from the need for children to develop skills to increase their independence in the adult world. Education is provided for about 12 years, but life goes on for decades after that.

Is the current education for children with disabilities beneficial, or are we simply distracted by the rhetoric and have lost our way? The reports to congress stress public schools complying with the law by showing 62% of special education students are spending most of their day in regular classrooms. This ignores the purpose of education to enable children to learn skills that help them function as an adult. The long-term goals should enable one to maintain focus on adult outcomes.

Research Based on High Functioning Children

Because the federal government requires education of disabled in regular classrooms, unless the school can justify the child's withdrawal from same, researchers choose higher functioning children as subjects, because they are easier to work with, they can function in a regular classroom, and they provide better outcomes. To ensure continued funding, researchers need to show positive results.

The research is based on the higher functioning subjects in the spectrum label and then is mistakenly applied to the lower functioning, thus misleading everyone into thinking that the teaching strategies are useful to all people with the label. This can result in false hopes and expectations on behalf of parents, who expect greater outcomes with strategies that actually don't apply to their children. Classic autism is rare and includes more severe communication difficulties and mental retardation. Therefore, teaching methods effective in higher functioning students are not necessarily appropriate for the rest of the spectrum.

Teaching Strategies Altered to fit the Regular Classroom

Since educational goals are determined by federal law to be disabled children learning in a regular classroom, the teaching strategies developed are based on this placement. But children with autism have difficulties generalizing information from the classroom to the real world. This lack of generalization was identified by Dr. Itard and Seguin two hundred years ago and they stated instruction must be given in the appropriate environment where the skill will be used. For example, instruction for setting the table and cooking should occur in the home and instruction on the use of transportation, recreation, and shopping occur in the community.

Dr. Temple Grandin has identified the lack of generalization when she writes in **Thinking in Pictures** (1995) *"A person with classic Kanner autism can be taught not to run out into the busy street in front of his house because it is dangerous. Unfortunately, he often fails to generalize this knowledge to a street at somebody else's house. In another scenario, the autistic person may learn the procedure for buying a candy bar at Safeway but* *have difficulty figuring out how to buy a candy bar at Walgreen's."* To properly address this difficulty with generalization, the child with autism has to be taught in a different manner and in different settings from typical children.

We know that children with autism have difficulties generalizing information from one environment to another, so how do researchers address this need? The National Research Council (2001) writes that the *"use of naturalistic teaching procedures" was "an attempt to improve generalization of skills to use in everyday life."* Yet the term "naturalistic teaching" simply refers to teaching strategies in a regular classroom. It does not refer to teaching skills in a variety of community environments where they are needed. The behavioral teaching strategies have been modified in an attempt to make them applicable in classes with typical peers.

A recently published book on training for generalization with *"science based best practices"* states that 1) using multiple examples of a concept (color, size) will increase the likelihood it will be generalized to other environments; and, 2) when conditions in the training setting are similar to the *"natural setting,"* generalization is more likely to occur. The contrived situation may seem similar to real life to a teacher, but not to the student, who is more attuned to details and differences. The teaching of skills needs to occur in the environment where the skill is useful for the student.

Although researchers recognize the problem of lack of generalization with children with autism and the need to teach in real world settings, the approach is to label the classroom as a "naturalistic environment." The goal has been changed from helping children with autism become more independent and self-sufficient as adults, to teaching them to function in a regular classroom. The strategies are structured to the placement and generalization is assumed by the use of a variety of materials, using different areas of the school and different people to provide the teaching. Generalization to the home and community is ignored, because that is not the goal of public education.

Researchers are not ignorant of the facts of lack of generalization, but choose to bend and twist the facts to meet their personal agenda: creating teaching strategies to be used in a classroom. The incentives to make decisions based on greater personal benefits override any decision that would benefit disabled children. The notion that creating a "natural environment" in the classroom will help generalize learning to the real-world is simply smoke and mirrors.

Researchers also transfer responsibility for education of children with autism to parents. The NRC writes that parents need to be involved in the education of their children in order to help children generalize information from the classroom to other environments.

Parents mistakenly think the school system is taking responsibility for providing an education that will enable children with autism to become more independent and self-sufficient as adults. In the 2011 Parade Magazine article on *Autism's Lost Generation,* one parent was quoted as saying *"You are devastated twice: first with the diagnosis; then, years later, when you realize that after all the interventions you still have a kid with autism and you have to plan his future."* The outcome is a needless and devastating blow to parents, who have been repeatedly told their children are making progress on their educational plans and implying that attending a regular class is a step toward normality.

Areas of Need Neglected

Adaptive behaviors are often deficient in children with autism, but educators tend to ignore these educational needs, because they are not taught in the regular classroom, and federal law requires education in the regular classroom. We can't expect adults with autism to become independent, if we don't get them out into the community, when they are children, to learn skills needed to function as adults.

In 2007, S. Williams White and colleagues published an article in the Journal of Autism and Developmental Disorders, stating *"Placement in regular education may inadvertently widen the gap in higher-functioning children if the teaching focus on traditional academics overshadows teaching other social and self-care skills these children need."* Unfortunately, the focus is still on children with autism functioning in a regular classroom and I do not expect this social perspective to change easily or quickly.

Others have recognized that current educational research ignores important areas, such as sensory issues, self-help skills, use of vigorous exercise, learning through reading and writing before speaking, use of music to teach language, teaching "to do" rather than "to know," but these aren't congruent with the federal law requiring education in the regular classroom. As a result, we have children leaving the school system without the ability to provide their own personal care, shop in a store, do their laundry, and cook their meals.

There are many areas of need that are not addressed, such as adaptive behaviors (life skills). Difficulties with adaptive behaviors are more predictive of future functioning than measurement of academic functioning (mental tests). Adaptive behavior refers to the life skills that people need to function independently, such as shopping, laundry, cleaning, cooking, and personal care such as eating, dressing, bathing, brushing teeth, hygiene, and toileting.

Educational Research lacks Validity

We have to be careful about drawing conclusions from scientific experiments. It is easy and even tempting to come to the premature conclusion of causation with the appearance of correlation – when two events occur in succession. We discussed this with the Lovaas study, when he tried to attribute the ABA method with higher IQ scores. Magical thinking and pseudoscience occur when we connect two successive events and conclude that the first event caused the second.

Correlation is a valuable type of scientific evidence in fields such as medicine, psychology, and sociology. But first, correlation must be confirmed as real, and then every possible causative relationship must be systematically explored. "Correlation is not causation" is a scientific principle.

The NRC wrote a chapter in **Educating Children with Autism** called "Methodological Issues in Research on Educational Interventions." They write that the interventions should demonstrate a causal relationship. It concerns me when educational researchers seem to be confusing correlation with causation. We can't begin to consider causation until studies are done comparing various interventions and that has not been done.

Educational Research being reviewed by peers before it is published in scientific publications is a problem, because it is confined to an internal circle of like-minded people. Standards for judging research should be beyond the control of peers. The National Research Council (NRC) reviewed ten

University based programs. Some of the programs reviewed were established and operated by members of the NRC, so in some cases, they were reviewing themselves.

The teachers who provide the instruction in an experimental study should not evaluate the progress of their students. The NRC acknowledges this *"potential effect of experimenter bias"* as most research today is violating good scientific practice, by allowing those involved in the research to collect the data. Are we are supposed to ignore the bad science and assume that these interventions should be used with our children, because a researcher claims they are "science-based best practices"?

When researchers publish study results, they refer to their study methods as "science-based best practices." Are these practices science-based? The lack of scientific evidence for these *"science-based best practices"* is well recognized. In 2011, a study was published in <u>Pediatrics</u> (Warren et al.) that reviewed 34 early intensive interventions for autism spectrum disorders. These were ABA based programs, including Lovaas and the Early Start Denver Model that are two of the model programs reviewed by the NRC. The authors found that *"Seventeen studies were case series; 2 were randomized controlled trials. Only 1 study was considered good and 23 were considered poor quality. The strength of the evidence ranged from insufficient to low."* Bad science does not allow one to make any valid conclusions and certainly any conclusions of causation would be highly premature and inappropriate.

After a review of the ten university based programs, the NRC stated that the research doesn't allow one to make a conclusion about the effectiveness of a given approach. So despite the lack of scientific evidence because of bad research, we are to take a giant leap and assume a majority of children participating in these research-based programs are making broad gains. In other words, despite the promotion of various approaches to treatment of children with autism as *"science based"* and *"best practices,"* there are no known effective treatments.

Experimental reproducibility is a major component of good science. In 2015, Roni Jacobson wrote an article in <u>Scientific American</u>, ***Massive International Project Raises Questions about the Validity of Psychology Research.*** He was reporting the results of a study that was published in the journal <u>Science</u> (Vol. 349, Issue 625i) that concluded only about 40 percent of the 100 experiments tested were replicable.

Dr. Flier, Dean of the Harvard Medical School, wrote a commentary article in the <u>Wall Street Journal</u> on March 2, 2016 called ***How to keep Bad Science from Getting into Print.*** He wrote that there was a *"retraction last August of 64 articles by one of the world's largest academic publishers, Springer,"* and the 1998 published paper claiming vaccines caused autism was retracted in 2010. The high number of retractions led to the widespread belief that results of studies are irreproducible.

Dr. Flier wrote that scientists may violate the scientific method because of the desire for career advancement and maintaining grant funding resulting in a considerable amount of junk science. It seems to be a conflict of interest for the Department of Education to fund research. The researcher depends on funding and cannot risk alienating the funding source with any outcomes that do not support the interests of the Department of Education.

With educational research depending on funding sources, we cannot expect good science. The focus becomes maintaining a funding source by giving positive results in order to support the professional's livelihood. There is no incentive for professionals to work together, to identify educational needs of children with autism, and how to properly educate children to become more independent and self-sufficient. It is my contention that we need to establish specialized schools for children with autism that are run by autism specialists trained in brain science to understand the learning needs and how to meet those needs, and include a curriculum for generalization of skills in various environments.

Who Benefits?

Are children with autism benefitting from fifty years of educational research and "science-based best practices"? If you want to know if the educational strategies are effective for children with autism, then you need to look at long-term outcomes. A 2015 report from the A.J. Drexel Autism Institute in Philadelphia stated that about 87 percent of young adults with autism live with a parent, compared to about 21 percent of all young adults. The lifetime cost of supporting an individual with autism is $2.4 million if the person has an intellectual disability, and at least 40 percent do, according to the report.

We already know that hundreds of thousands of children with autism are leaving the school system without the ability to take care of their own needs, so they require lifetime care. This is similar to the actions of psychiatrists, who ignored the long-term outcome for lobotomies that resulted in families caring for their loved ones. It is easy to show short-term gains in academic work that is meaningless in the long-term.

Education has failed our children. Yet, we continue to make the same mistakes. Despite the poor long-term outcomes, we cling to the belief that people with disabilities simply need opportunities to learn. This has resulted in treating adults with disabilities as if they have just not received enough education. For example, adults with disabilities attend day programs that require educational classes for the rest of their lives. The funding sources for the day programs require the classes based on the old idea that education can cure disabilities. Therefore, we have adults attending classes in day programs throughout their adult lives. We continue the belief despite outcomes that demonstrate the fallacy of our system. Rather than treating adults with disabilities with respect and dignity, we force them to continue education for the rest of their lives, in a classroom that fails to meet their needs.

The teachers of these adult educational programs often have no training in special needs, as we seem to think that anyone can teach a child with disabilities. In one class I observed, the teacher was talking about telling time. She drew a circle on the board with the numbers and hands of the clock. She had handouts with pictures of clocks showing different times and the students were to mark the correct times as shown on the clocks. Unfortunately, most of the adult students in the room could not count to 12 and did not understand the concept of one-quarter or one-half.

Wouldn't it make more sense to provide structured opportunities for exercise, crafts, games, and accessing various community environments rather than continuation of useless academic classes?

Model Programs and Public Education

Research is conducted within model programs consisting of highly trained staff specialized in autism. The National Research Council reports on the ten programs representing research in autism stating *"All ten programs are directed by at least one doctoral level professional with a long-standing reputation in the treatment of autistic spectrum disorders. In addition, virtually every program developer is assisted by either doctoral or master's-level personnel ...In almost all of the programs, college students play key roles in their service delivery systems."* In other words, these model programs are not comparable to a typical public school classroom, where the teacher may have no knowledge of autism spectrum disorders, and they do not have the low student-teacher ratio present in the model programs.

Autism researchers and specialists at the university level do not typically teach undergraduates, since the competition for tenure revolves around research and publication. The National Research Council reports *"personnel preparation remains one of the weakest elements of effective programming for children with autistic spectrum disorders and their families. There is a short supply of expertise and experience in the field of education for children with autistic spectrum disorders and special attention should be paid to rapidly increase the capabilities of the trainers, who may have experience in special education or related fields, but not in the special skills and practices for children with autistic spectrum disorders."* All this great funding for research and education has yet to result in public school special education teachers trained to work with children with autism spectrum disorders.

The National Research Council writes that many of the research developed teaching strategies are not well known to parents or professionals. They state *"Newer behavioral approaches such as incidental teaching and pivotal response training stress naturalistic delivery, are used in group settings, and allow easier coordination with inclusion ... but are not as well known to the public, either parents or professionals."* A 2015 article in the Journal of Autism and Developmental Disorders by Shreibman, Dawson and colleagues wrote that they had made progress in developing teaching strategies but *"they are not yet widely delivered in community settings thus limiting the range of types of intervention available to children and families."* The NRC states *"The national challenge is to close the gap between the quality of model programs and the reality of most publicly funded early educational programs."*

Many of the teaching interventions developed within the framework of ABA, are complex. For example, the NRC reports that to prepare peers to interact with children with autism requires *"socially skilled typical peers and precise adult control during training of peers, managing and fading reinforcement, and monitoring ongoing child interaction data."* Behavioral approaches generally demand considerable data collection. Shreibman and colleagues (2015) state *"Data collection is a critical aspect to any approach based in ABA."* That works for researchers, but isn't very practical for parents and educators.

Teaching strategies are made more complex because of the creation of new terminology (psychobabble) that must be mastered by parents and educators to try to understand the techniques. Psychologists love to create new terms for their theories, such as *"environmental stimuli," "cues," "prompts," "discrimination training," "shaping and fading," "naturalistic interventions," "antecedents and consequences," "aversives," "scaffolding," "differential reinforcement," "discriminative stimulus"*, and the list can go on forever. Recently, I read an article on teaching strategies that referred to parents as *"natural change agents"* LOL!

When researchers become too removed from the real world of teachers working in the trenches, one has to wonder if the teaching strategies created could actually be implemented in a regular classroom where the student-teacher ratio is not likely to approach 1:1. Many of the strategies require teachers to arrange a context in which to create an opportunity to teach a skill, and this may not be realistic for a teacher with many students of varying abilities. What teacher is going to have the time or inclination to create special situations for teaching one student in a regular classroom, when she/he may have no understanding of the needs of children with autism?

Are special education teachers trained to work with children with autism spectrum disorders? Dr. Candace Baker in <u>Special Education Journal</u> states, *"Currently, most undergraduate teacher preparation programs in higher education offer training as a generalist special education teacher."* Using Barnhill, Polloway, and Sumutka (2011) survey of 87 institutions of higher learning, Dr. Baker reported their survey *"showed that 41% of reporting institutions offered no ASD-specific coursework within the special education degree. In addition, half of the institutions indicated their states had not developed autism competencies for educators, 30% said their states did have autism competencies, and 14% did not know whether their state had competencies for autism."* If the special education teachers are not qualified, then one has to question the ability of aides in the classroom to understand how to provide an effective educational program for children with autism.

The NRC writes that parents need training about autism and treatments for autism *"to ensure that skills learned in the education program transfer to the home setting and to teach their child the many behaviors that are best mastered in the home and community."* If teachers are not properly trained in the condition of autism and teaching strategies, then how are they going to train parents?

There seem to be plenty of educational researchers telling others what to do, as long as they don't have to do it, and don't have to take responsibility for the outcomes. The only people who seem to benefit from "science-based best practices" are the researchers of these model programs. The funding for research does not include training teachers in the public schools. Many of the model programs will provide training in public schools, but at a very high price. Once site stated that it would be up to $2,000 for one trainer to come into the public school for one day, and the cost was considerably higher for more trainers over a longer period of time.

Secrets Revealed

The government funding for research for autism began in the 1960's and created a vast industry of educational researchers competing for grants. Publication of their research is referred to as *"science based best practices."* The label is impressive, but misleading. There is no research comparing teaching strategies to demonstrate best practices.

Researchers have a vested interest in promoting their work as successful, even when it fails to meet the needs of children with autism. The strategies are altered to meet the needs of the federal Government and those providing the grants. The focus is on short-term goals to show some sort of achievement, and ignores the long-term goals of adult independence and self-sufficiency. Despite fifty years of research, we are not obtaining the results needed by individuals with autism. Most of the research labs are based on behavioral theory that everything can be taught and this ignores brain science.

The goal for our children is to become adults who can function in a variety of community environments as independently as possible. A child attends a classroom for only a few years, compared to the rest of his life in the real world. The measure of success is not attendance in a regular classroom, but progression toward independent functioning. Does your child's program include daily exercise, hobbies, structured social activities, good manners, functional communication and independence in daily activities? Don't worry about your child having a job, if he can't take care of his personal needs, cook a meal and do his laundry.

Parents and teachers have been led to believe that attendance in a regular classroom makes the child higher functioning than children in a special education classroom. The real test is the level of independence the child can achieve as an adult to access a variety of environments and achieve a quality life.

The National Research Council (2001) writes: *"Some drawbacks, when looking at education of children with autism, involve the fact that these children do not demonstrate typical patterns of development in several key areas (communication, language and speech development, social development). Nor do they necessarily learn through developmentally typical teaching practices (verbal instruction, imitation of teachers and peers, and independent learning), because these strategies are often dependent on a child's internal motivation to learn, to be like others, and to gain competence."* The NRC seems to blame the child for failing to learn in the regular classroom due to "lack of motivation." Despite the identification of these teaching difficulties, educators continue to compare children with autism with children who follow a typical developmental pattern, and then try to teach them to learn like typical children in a regular classroom. If a child with autism is only compared to normal development and we fail to understand the neurological impairment, we only teach to the deficit and fail to accommodate the deficit. When educators assume children with autism process information the same as typical children, then they fail to understand how they think and learn differently. It is time to reveal these mistakes and learn how children with autism think and learn differently, so they must be taught differently.

Polly Yarnall, autism educational consultant, writes that *"automatic inclusion violates spirit and letter of IDEA; opportunities for successful inclusion begin to plateau by end of third grade as work becomes more abstract and faster paced; increasing use of language-based instruction puts students with autism at great disadvantage; sensory and processing difficulties tend to be insufficiently accommodated; regular education setting not necessarily best learning environment for students with autism; teachers and students in inclusion classrooms are typically ill prepared to receive student."* She also states that errors with inclusion include *"providing insufficient training, preparation, information, and support to personnel; placing student in settings where level of auditory and visual stimulation is typically too intense; assigning student work in which cognitive demands exceed student's ability to comprehend; depending on support of 1:1 aide; maintaining placement in face of frequent or severe disruptive behaviors; focusing on academics to detriment or exclusion of functional competencies; not offering multiple opportunities to apply functional skills.*

Parents of higher functioning children often report they wish they had spent more time on functional living skills. Sometimes we get distracted and establish goals for our children that meet our needs or the teacher's needs, more than the child's needs. For example, parents and teachers often want the child to have social conversations and friendships, while the child's needs are to learn to function in structured social environments.

The school system separates children based on age and speaks of "age appropriate activities" for our children with autism. Our children are then placed in a classroom with children who are the same chronological age, but have different needs. Age appropriate activities are developed for the learning needs of typical children, and not the needs of children with autism.

Don't get mislead by the idea that children with autism should attend a classroom based on age. It can be very beneficial to have our children attend a classroom with younger children. If you find a good classroom teacher or teacher's aide and your child is thriving, consider extending the placement based on the child's needs, not his age. I found a community preschool class that was small and had a teacher who worked well with David. She wasn't trained to work with special needs children, but she was well organized and the class was structured. She was a former singer and would sing instructions to David. We worked well together and maintained close communication. It worked so well, David stayed in her class until he was seven years old and thrived from the experience.

As a teenager, David was on a gymnastics team of boys that were five years younger than he was. It didn't bother David and he experienced success with an activity that he could participate in. As an adult, he has attended a water aerobics for ten years with mainly senior aged women. They love his enthusiasm and he thrives on the structure. He enjoys being around other people, without the pressure of trying to participate in a social conversation.

The next section will reveal the secrets of brain science that can connect brain structure and function to the behaviors in autism.

Section Two: Brain Function in Autism

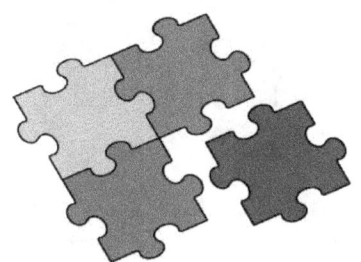

Chapter 6

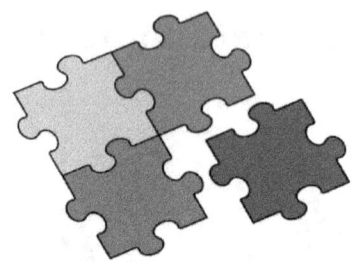

Sensations and Perceptions

The eye only sees what the brain is prepared to comprehend.
Henri Bergson or Robertson Davies.

Sensation and perception are different. Sensation refers to sensing our environment through sound, sight, touch, taste and smell. Perception involves judgment and interpretation of the world rather than a passive reaction to sensory input. It relies on brain function. We often assume that everyone feels and understands sensations in the same manner, but this is not true.

Temple Grandin writes in **The Way I See It** (2008) *"Children and adults with autism spectrum disorders, be they mildly or severely challenged, have one or more of their senses affected to the extent that it interferes with their ability to learn and process information from the world around them."* We should consider behaviors in autism as indicative of different sensory and perceptive processing. Drs. Itard and Seguin felt sensory processing was the core feature and some authors with ASD (e.g. T. Grandin; G. Gerland; J. Sinclair; D. Williams) report that autism is related to sensory processing.

Lovaas reported that in his 1987 experiment that the children who "recovered" all imitated speech within three months of starting the ABA program and those children who did not improve were visual learners. This clearly recognizes that some children with autism have stronger visual processing and some have stronger auditory processing.

We don't describe blind children by their behaviors, such as repetitive head movements, lack of eye contact, and touching objects because we recognize they have sensory processing difficulties. Yet, we describe behaviors in children with autism as "repetitive and stereotyped" and judge it as bizarre, then try to teach them to "act normal." It is time we considered that children with autism are "blind but can see" and "deaf but can hear."

Sounds

Although the child with autism can hear and see, his brain may not interpret the incoming sensations. Professionals repeatedly point out that a child with autism doesn't respond to many sounds, but obviously can hear, because he will run to the sound of removing paper from a familiar candy. This reflects the association of meaning with the sound from the child's perspective. The child is familiar with the sound of the paper being removed from something he likes and he runs to it.

My son, David, would suddenly run into the room when the TV played one of his favorite commercials. Therefore, hearing is excellent when associated with something meaningful to the child. This means the brain connected the sensation with a meaning or interpretation only when it had special meaning to the child. It is difficult for us to take a different perspective because our brains are wired differently.

Sometimes children with autism respond to sounds in a manner we consider socially inappropriate. When I took David into a public restroom, if it had an electric hand dryer and someone turned it on, he would try to crawl up the walls. He didn't understand the sound and he didn't observe others using the hand dryer to associate a meaning to the sound. Once I taught him how to use the hand dryer, he had control over the sound and it created meaning for him and he behaved appropriately.

There are many sounds in a home that a child with autism can have difficulty with, such as a vacuum cleaner or blender. Once the child is taught to use the item, he can connect meaning to the object, and this usually eliminates aberrant behavior. For example, the child can learn to vacuum while using earplugs or while listening to music.

Drs. Itard and Seguin discovered that when a child does not observe and imitate, then they have to be taught the use of objects in the environment where it would be used. This enables the child to connect meaning (purpose) with the use of objects. Temple Grandin writes in **The Autistic Brain** (2014) *"I've heard a lot of people with autism say that if they can initiate the sound, they're more likely to be able to tolerate it. The same is true if they know the sound is coming."*

We have to consider every environment from the autistic child's perspective. He does not understand the sights and sounds and this can be very distressing. When David was 12, he went to a skating rink where a friend was having a birthday party. Since typical children enjoy intense sensory input, the rink had music, a disco light, and video games. It was busy with children moving around and making lots of noise. David started skating and the lighting suddenly dimmed. He sat down confused. In a few moments, he started skating again. There were several times he sat down when the lighting or music changed. He was focused on skating and all this extraneous input was confusing.

David loves video games, so after skating, he started playing games. Several children were watching him and suddenly, I saw him try to push a child away. I knew it was time to leave. By the time I got him into the car, he was banging his head against the door. Being in a strange environment with lots of auditory and visual stimulation can be challenging and exhausting to an autistic child who doesn't understand the intense sensory input in an environment. The constant unexpected environmental assaults on his nervous system will result in behavior meltdowns.

When typical people hear sudden, unusual noises, we stop, look and listen to try to attach meaning to the sound. It is the fight or flight response to possible danger. When an autistic person reacts to a sudden noise, such as a blender or electric hand dryer, with screaming and trying to get away from the sound, we label the behavior as "over-reaction to loud sounds." We cannot interpret behaviors of children with sensory processing disorders as if they should react like neurotypicals (NT).

What if we tried to understand behaviors from a biological perspective? If the brain can't connect meaning with the incoming information then the body would react with stress. Cortisol released during stress affects brain cells by allowing more calcium to enter the cells. In the short term, it helps the cells stay active to respond to danger. In the long term, cells can become overloaded with calcium, so they fire too frequently and die.

Cognitive symptoms of stress include inability to focus, worrying, forgetfulness, agitation, moodiness, avoiding others and feeling overwhelmed. Some of the physical symptoms include rapid heartrate, high blood pressure, headaches and ringing in the ears. The National Research Council published **Educating Children with Autism,** where they wrote about a study that showed *"a tendency toward cortisol hypersecretion during school hours was found, and it appeared to be an environmental stress response (Richdale and Prior, 1992)."* Viewed from this perspective, David's stress experience in the skating rink begins to make sense. It is better to try to understand behavior, rather than label behavior aberrant and attempt to extinguish it.

Can you imagine the stress for a young child with autism in a classroom environment with all the bewildering incoming sensations? He will have difficulties knowing what to focus on and how to interpret what he sees and hears. If he can't process words and gestures at the same time, he may end up with a meltdown. It is a mistake to interpret behaviors in children with autism as a desire for attention, an attempt to avoid a task, or a communication problem when that is seldom a reflection of how the child responds to the environment.

Vision

We attend to what the brain processes as important in the environment, so if the brain does not attach significance to various aspects of the environment, then we ignore it. The behavior of children with autism who often focus on a small detail, such as a crack in the floor or piece of string, indicates they connect meaning to things we don't understand. Patients with brain damage can often help us understand how someone can see, but not connect meaning to what they see.

Dr. V.S. Ramachandran in **The Tell-Tale Brain** (2011) writes about a patient who had a stroke resulting in retaining the ability to identify shapes and lines and the relationship between them, but lost the ability to process additional meaning to what was seen. The condition is called "agnosia" where the patient can see, but doesn't know what he sees. It can result in strange behaviors, such as described by Dr. Ramachandran about his patient: *"He could trim hedges with shears or pull out a plant from the*

*soil. And yet he could not tell weeds from flowers, or for that matter recognize
faces or cars or tell salad dressing from cream. Thus symptoms that would
otherwise seem bizarre and incomprehensible begin to make sense in terms of
(brain function)."* An individual can have sight, but still be unable to identify
what he is seeing.

In Chapter one, I discussed how Dr. Itard had taught Victor to
identify various objects in Victor's room, but when the same objects were on a
table in Dr. Itard's office, Victor could not identify them. The items were
clearly visible to Victor, but he could not identify them.

The condition of agnosia helps explain some of David's strange
behaviors. David can draw, but often does not know what he is drawing. For
example, he drew a dog with a collar, but colored both the same color. When I
told him the collar was a decoration and could be colored differently, he was
surprised. He attends to the lines of an object without knowing what he is
drawing, because his brain does not automatically interpret meaning to what
is being drawn.

David attended an art class, where they were to draw a skeleton
placed in front of the room. David was the only student to draw the metal rod
holding the skeleton together. He was not able to make a judgment or
interpretation of the metal rod as separate from the skeleton and having the
purpose of holding the bones together.

David does not draw from memory, but only from a picture or object
placed in front of him. Dr. Ramachandran wrote about his patient that *"one
of the most intriguing symptoms became manifest when he was asked to draw
flowers from memory."* The patient drew flowers and labeled them, but he
was unaware that they did not resemble real flowers. We are not talking
about a language problem, but a perceptual problem. The brain can process
what it sees, but also needs to interpret meaning to what it sees.

The brain is normally designed to enable us to make a judgment or
interpretation to what we see beyond line, color, or motion. This requires
extensive connections throughout the brain. We often think of the brain
processing vision in only one area of the brain, but there are at least thirty
areas that are required to process vision and this does not include
interpreting meaning to what we see.

Children with autism sometimes have a stress (fearful) reaction to what they see. Charles Hart in **Without Reason** (1989) wrote about his son's fear of shower curtains. Since we observe the environment and interpret meaning to what we see, we have great difficulty understanding the autistic perspective. The child can see, but may not be able to interpret what he sees. Perhaps it is viewed as a wall that suddenly moves. Perhaps it has a strange print or design. Perhaps it makes a noise when you move it. The challenge is to try to understand how the curtain might be perceived by the child and how to make it meaningful to the child. Although we easily understand the purpose or social intent of the shower curtain, the child does not. If the child has not encountered it before, and does not understand its purpose, it could be frightening.

David and I were in the swimming pool when he was four years old. We went twice a week, and often counted jumps into the water from the side of the pool, then I pulled him through the water. One day, as I was moving him through the water, he suddenly became upset and was pulling away. I moved away from the spot where the fear reaction started and explored the area. There was a drain on the bottom of the pool that was distinctly different from the smooth surface elsewhere. Autistics focus on differences and this visual difference on the bottom of the pool surface was disturbing him. I approached the drain, but kept him away from it. I stepped on the drain as he was looking at it. Once I acknowledged the visual difference, the fear subsided. If the brain does not have the connections to interpret what is seen then a fear reaction can be expected.

Brain research reveals that autistics focus on one detail in the environment and fail to distinguish what is important from what is irrelevant. "Importance" suggests "meaning" and the child with ASD does not process meaning with what he sees. It takes patience to look for the one detail in the environment that the child is responding to and try to accommodate that focus, before trying to push the child to focus on what we may consider important.

We were attending a Boy Scout Christmas party being held in the school cafeteria. David, age eight, and my husband, Jerry, were sitting at a table, while I was talking with someone in another part of the room. Suddenly, out of the corner of my eye, I saw David running. He was running into people! He ran into three people before I got to him. I grabbed him and said, "*Stop.*" In a few moments, I felt his body relax and we walked back to the table.

Jerry was wiping a spill that had occurred at the table. Apparently, he spilled a drink and left to go find some paper towels. When David noticed the spill, he started to run. We don't know how David perceived the liquid flowing across the table. Was the table melting? We cannot assume that an autistic child can understand the environment the way we do. We can't assume that David understood what he saw at the table. If we focus only on the running behavior, then we may not understand the problem from the child's perspective.

Motion

We do not see with our eyes; we see with our brains. It is the brain that interprets all the sensory information into meaning. The eyes don't take a picture. The brain scatters incoming information (motion, color, depth, lines, etc.) to various areas of the brain to be processed. There are messages going back and forth to different areas. If the brain is able to process all parts of vision, then we will perceive an accurate result. But that is not always the case.

One aspect of vision is motion. The ability to detect motion is vital to survival – to avoid the snake in the grass or something flying through the air. Although autistics often develop fear of unusual objects, they are sometimes described as "*having no fear.*" Typically, we attend to sudden motion that might indicate danger. If we are trying to detect the presence of someone in a dark room, we seek signs of motion. Perhaps if the brain does not associate motion with fear, then autistics would not show fear with motion.

What would sight be like if we could not detect movement? Dr. Oliver Sacks described a patient who had a stroke in the visual cortex of her brain and it affected her ability to see motion. She could not cross the street, because she did not see the cars moving. She saw a series of static pictures. Therefore, she could not tell how fast the car was approaching. In addition, talking to people was difficult because she could not see changing facial expressions. Since she had years of experience seeing motion, she was aware she had lost this ability.

Temple Grandin in Thinking in Pictures that she *"loved to spin and seldom got dizzy. When I stopping spinning, I enjoyed the sensation of the room spinning."* David would spin himself when he was in a swimming pool. Although we tried to teach him to use a swing, he always preferred lying across the seat of the swing and spinning. If you spin yourself, the world would be seen in motion. Often children with autism like to spin themselves and they do not get dizzy like typical children – unless they are ill.

Children with autism also like some things that move, such as ceiling fans. Temple Grandin writes about her interest in automatic sliding doors and the thrill it gave her when the movement of the door crossed her eyes. David would squeal with laughter when watching a little toy car move across the track. Often a child with autism will stare out the side window of a moving car with great delight. Would flicking fingers by the eyes create a sense of motion?

Internal Body Sensations

The hypothalamus is the brain's master regulatory structure. It affects the function of many internal organs, regulating body temperature, body rhythms, blood pressure, and blood glucose levels. It is also involved in regulating thirst, hunger, aggression and lust. From birth, David displayed a variety of difficulties with perceiving internal body sensations, such as hunger, thirst, body temperature and need to have a bowel movement. He did not cry from hunger, so I fed him on a schedule. This inability of my son to interpret sensations has resulted in numerous challenging situations.

I encountered a problem of David rubbing his forehead across the carpet and creating a bruise on his forehead. Knowing that people often get headaches when they are dehydrated, I increased his intake of fluids and it resolved the problem. David still does not respond to thirst, so he was taught to have something to drink after exercise, working in the yard, or being outside in hot weather. If someone observed him having a drink after working in the yard, they would not be aware of his sensory deficit and that this was a routine created for him to adapt to his lack of thirst. By giving David a rule to have eight glasses of fluid per day, he counts the number of glasses he drinks every day.

Another area where David had difficulty interpreting sensations was the need to have a bowel movement. He was five years old and had been trained to urinate in the toilet by including trips to the toilet during his daily routines. He was not bowel trained and like many children with ASD, he had very large bowel movements. They are often diagnosed with a mega colon (large colon) perhaps because they do not interpret the sensation properly and go to the bathroom in a timely manner.

I decided to try an experiment (this is not intended as medical advice!). I gave David a Fleet's enema. He held on for forty-five minutes. He would lie on the floor for a few minutes and then I would put him back on the toilet. Finally, he let go and had a bowel movement in the toilet. I directed his attention to what he had done and congratulated him. I waited two weeks and did it again. He held on for fifteen minutes and then pooped in the toilet. He was toilet trained. My theory is that he could not interpret the body sensation, so he held on rather than letting go, thus creating a large colon.

David often has difficulty adapting to changes in temperature. When the weather turned cold, he wore a sweatshirt to gymnastics class. I discovered he would not take the sweatshirt off once he started exercising, so we had to create a routine of taking his sweatshirt off, before he started class. Now, David checks the outdoor thermometer before going out, to determine if he should put a jacket on. We also have to remind him when the weather changes to start wearing long pants and shirts, and stop wearing shorts and light shirts.

There have been case reports that behaviors of children with autism may improve with fever. For example, a study was published by Curran and colleagues in 2007 called *Behaviors Associated with Fever in Children with Autism Spectrum Disorders (ASD).* The authors studied 30 children (aged 2-18 years) with autism during and after an episode of fever by collecting parent responses to the Aberrant Behavior Checklist. The results were that fewer aberrant behaviors recorded on the subscales of irritability, hyperactivity, stereotypy, and inappropriate speech compared with control subjects. The authors concluded there was behavior change during fever, but they still could not state the underlying brain mechanisms for it. I have observed the same effect on my son, David. In addition, David could not spin when he had a temperature, because he would get dizzy. In other words, he had a normal reaction to spinning when he was febrile.

Taste and Smell

Many children with autism like to smell things and may identify people and things through smell. In addition, many children with autism find certain textures, tastes and smells of food unappealing. David doesn't like the texture of a tomato, but likes the taste when cooked in sauce. He also has difficulty with spicy foods.

In *Chapter One*, **The Forgotten Past**, I discussed how Dr. Itard taught to the senses. He reported that Victor did not like sweets like most children. He had Victor sample and differentiate an acid liquid (pickle juice) from a sweet liquid. When Dr. Itard began teaching Victor to perceive different tastes, he noted this enabled Victor to eat other foods that he had always avoided.

Pain and Touch

Children with autism often have a different (less than expected) reaction to pain. When my son, David, was less than a year old, I noticed he had one eye shut. He did not cry or try to touch the eye. After taking him for a medical examination, I discovered he had a severe corneal abrasion. He may have scratched his eye with his fingernail. I encountered numerous occasions where David demonstrated strange behaviors to physical symptoms.

One day, I saw David rubbing his hand on the grass. My first interpretation was thinking about our dog and David may have put his hand in dog poop. I went to investigate and discovered he had burned his hand on the grill. He felt something, but did not know what it meant and did not associate emotion with the event.

Typical children learn to seek comfort when they are hurt so Mom can kiss it and make it better, or put a bandage on it. They also learn to exaggerate an injury to get attention from Mom. Children with autism don't associate these emotions with an injury and don't seek comfort. David could be cut and bleeding and he didn't seem to notice. Even as an adult, he does not flinch when getting a shot, getting blood drawn or having a splinter removed.

Dr. Ramachandran in **The Tell-Tale Brain** (2011) writes about a patient who could feel pain, but would respond with laughter. He stated that a CT (computed tomography) scan *"revealed that one of the pain pathways in her brain was damaged."* Pain is initially processed in an area beneath the temporal lobe and then travels to an area in the frontal lobes where emotion and danger are processed. There are patients who do not have this secondary connection to the frontal lobes so they feel pain, but do not interpret the sensation or add meaning to it.

Processing sensations and perceptions requires extensive connections throughout the brain and these connections are deficient in autism. For example, David was five years old and I was trying to toilet train him for bowel movements. He was sitting on the toilet and started to scream. I discovered his wool shirt was hitting his leg. When I removed the shirt, he stopped screaming, but when it hit his leg, he screamed. I was baffled, because he felt the sensation, but he didn't try to push the shirt away. He failed to connect the shirt with feeling something on his leg.

Touch can be a pleasant or unpleasant sensation. When David was a baby, he pulled away from a light touch, but enjoyed deep pressure. For many years, he would seek this pressure sensation by crawling under sofa cushions, or a mattress. He also seemed to like the washer during the spin cycle and the dryer when it was operating. Rather than extinguishing the behaviors, we tried to assist him in achieving something that was calming to him. We bought a vibrator that we used on his back, arms and legs and he loved it.

Temple Grandin developed her squeeze machine to help calm her body by providing and controlling touch. She wrote how people in her life tried to prevent her use of the squeeze machine, because of their subjective judgment that it was weird or inappropriate behavior. Before we start to extinguish behavior, we need to examine it from the child's perspective and what purpose it serves him or her.

David loved soft, furry things and one year, he made this explicitly clear to us. We were at the mall, and he ran to a woman in a fur coat and hugged the coat – much to the woman's displeasure! He also would bury his head in a table of sweaters and anyone who wore a soft sweater could find herself on the receiving end of David's head on her sweater. The challenge was finding ways he could enjoy the sensations in a socially appropriate manner. David's focus was on one detail – the softness of materials.

I went to a fabric store and purchased a soft piece of fabric with polka dots (he loved polka dots). After his bath, he was wrapped in this fabric and he clearly loved the sensation. I then took a small piece of the fabric and when we went to the mall, I put the piece of fabric in his hand and told him it was his fabric. When we went by the sweater table, I stopped him from grabbing sweaters and showed him the fabric in his hand. There are methods of helping the child meet his needs in socially appropriate ways. It isn't always a matter of extinguishing behaviors, but altering the behavior to meet the child's needs and make it more socially acceptable.

When David was "graduating" from preschool, the students were all going to wear paper graduation hats, but David would take his hat off and throw it on the ground. Rather than viewing the behavior as typical childhood defiance, we always have to try to view the experience from the child's sensory deficits. David would wear a baseball cap, so we stapled the graduation hat onto the baseball cap and he wore it with no problems.

Secrets Revealed

When behaviors can be associated with how the child senses and processes his environment, then they begin to make sense. Rather than describe behaviors as "restricted and repetitive" or as "doesn't pay attention," or as "hypo- or hyper- sound sensitivities, we need to interpret the behaviors in terms of how the child learns and this results from brain structure and function in autism.

We know that people with autism report that if they can initiate a sound or know the sound is coming, they are more likely to tolerate it. Rather than describe behaviors as hypo- or hyper-response to sounds, it is more beneficial to understand how to help people with autism adjust to sounds in the environment. Most people react with a flight or fight response to unusual or unfamiliar sounds. We have to determine if the sound (e.g. gunshot, lightening) might indicate danger. When a child with autism reacts to sound with a fight or flight response, we need to convey the meaning or purpose of the sound to a child and then they are able to have a more acceptable response.

A study of children with autism in school demonstrated increased cortisol secretions indicating an environmental stress response. We need to recognize sensory processing abnormalities in children with autism and help them cope with these problems. We can't expect them to "act normal" when their brains do not process the environment in the typical manner.

We often think of a brain abnormality as "all or nothing" and don't recognize that the problem can be related to the brain only partially processing a sensation. We have to consider that children with autism may be "blind but can see" and "deaf but can hear." In Chapter one, Dr. Itard reported that Victor could not identify the objects on the table in his office that were clearly visible to him and these were items he had previously identified in his bedroom. In neurology, there is a condition called "agnosia" where the patient can see, but doesn't know what he sees.

Children with autism lack long distance connections in the brain that enable them to properly interpret what they see, hear, feel, taste and smell. Therefore, their behaviors reflect this brain abnormality and must be accommodated. This is discussed in more detail in the next chapter.

In the next chapter, we will examine brain science that demonstrates that behaviors in autism are related to the lack of pretend play and exploratory play, lack of facial identification, lack of social interaction, and inability to combine details with main concept.

Chapter 7

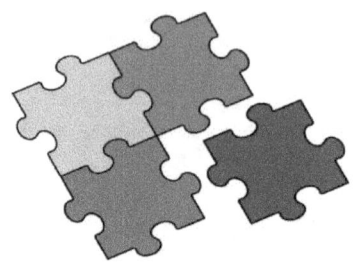

Brain Function and Autism
We will understand autism only when we understand the brain. Cheryl Merritt

For most of the twentieth century, human behavior was defined by environmental theories, such as Freud with psychoanalysis, Skinner with behaviorism, and education with Piaget's stages of development. These theories all relied on the idea that babies are born as blank slates and we teach them everything they know. But now we know better.

Temple Grandin in **The Autistic Brain** (2014) writes, *"Thanks to advances in neuroscience and genetics, we can begin phase three in the history of autism."* She writes that we can now search for causes with observable neurological and genetic evidence based on each symptom. In this chapter, I will connect behaviors in autism with the structure and function in the brain that result in these behaviors. Once we understand these symptoms from a brain function perspective, we can develop teaching strategies for the individual.

Starting in the 1990's – the decade of the brain – neuroscience accomplished amazing things and is finally able to explain learning differences in autism based on brain research. The research takes multiple different perspectives – genetic, cellular, post mortem, split brain patients, brain imaging, and study of patients with brain deficits. We can begin to put the autism puzzle together by examining the various avenues of research on the brain as it relates to behaviors seen in autism. If we only discussed one approach we could not obtain a complete picture.

We will examine the various areas of brain deficits in children with autism as revealed by brain research and connect it to the symptoms of autism, including lack of observation and imitation, lack of pretend play, language and social communication problems, and repetitive behaviors.

Mirror Neuron System

As often happens, discoveries are made by accident. In the 1990's, Rizzolatti and colleagues were investigating individual brain cells (motor) in monkeys. Electrodes were on specific brain cells to monitor its activity when it picked up something to eat. One day, a researcher walked into the laboratory and picked up a raisin and ate it. The monitor for the monkey's brain cell buzzed! It appeared that the brain cells responded to the observation of others eating a raisin. This was the beginning of an extraordinary discovery that when we observe someone doing something, our brains react as if we are doing it ourselves, even when we are not making the movement. This instinctual behavior to observe and imitate is part of the brain structure present in babies and is referred to as "mirror neurons," because these are brain cells that enable us to mirror behaviors we observe in others.

Although this study was on individual neurons, we are actually talking about a mirror neuron system, because these neurons are located in different areas and are connected to many other areas (structures) of the brain. Since this initial research, scientists have conducted more studies on normal and autistic children using various brain imaging techniques confirming the mirror neuron system dysfunction in children with autism, resulting in a lack of ability to observe and imitate.

Dr. Ramachandran and colleagues used an electroencephalogram (EEG) measurement of brain waves showing a component called the "mu wave" is blocked anytime a person makes a voluntary muscle movement. It is also blocked when a person observes someone else perform the same movement. When the first child with autism was tested, they stated *"The EEG showed that the child had an observable mu wave that was suppressed when he made a simple voluntary movement, just as in normal children. But when the child watched someone else perform the action, the suppression did not occur. We concluded that the child's motor command system was intact but that his mirror neuron system was deficient."* This study was followed up with a study of ten children with autism showing the same results.

Other researchers have confirmed these results using different brain imaging techniques – magnetoencephalography, which measures the magnetic field produced by electric current in the brain, functional magnetic resonance imaging, and transcranial magnetic stimulation. These studies provide compelling evidence that children with autism spectrum disorders have **Dysfunctional Mirror Neuron Systems.**

First, let's compare normal functioning with this brain deficit. In the 1970's, Meltzoff did a study that demonstrated newborns imitate an adult making faces, such as sticking out her tongue, within the first hour of birth. We don't teach a baby to imitate, because they are born with brains designed to learn by observation and imitation. By three months of age, babies have the ability to follow a person's eye gaze, as well as mimic any emotion in the face.

Children with autism have difficulties with observation and imitation. I viewed a videotape of elementary children with autism following a leader doing calisthenics at the Higashi School in Japan. Some of the children would only move one arm or one leg or only move the upper part of the body. The students would tend to one detail, but fail to process the whole movement. The teachers came up behind the children and helped them by putting their bodies through the motions. Even though the children could see the leader, they were unable to observe and imitate. Neuroscience has finally explained this brain deficit.

Charles Hart wrote in **Without Reason** (1989) about his autistic son, Ted, attending a birthday party where they had ice cream cones. Ted simply let the ice cream melt and run down his fingers, because he had never had ice cream in a cone. He had always eaten it in a dish. Ted did not observe and imitate the other children eating ice cream cones because of this mirror neuron system deficit.

In *Chapter 1*, **The Forgotten Past**, Drs. Itard and Seguin in the 1800's discussed the difficulty of teaching children with autism because of their lack of observation and imitation. It took almost two centuries for neurologists to prove it is a neurological deficit.

How the Brain Interprets Meaning

When we observe and imitate others, it isn't just "monkey see; monkey do." The brain processes meaning to what we observe. In normal development, imitation results from observing others and attaching meaning to what we observe. This is how the brain typically works to help the child create an understanding of the world. When children have a pretend tea party or pretend to cook something, they have to understand the meaning of the behavior. It isn't just imitating motions; it is incorporating meaning or social intent to motions. It is the brain that enables us to connect meaning to everything we see, such as play behaviors, facial expressions and emotions, words and gestures.

The brain has complex anatomy and function. The cerebrum makes up about three-fourths of the total volume of the brain. It is divided into the right and left hemispheres connected by a large trundle of nerve fibers (wires) called the corpus callosum. This connection is necessary because the two hemispheres need to communicate extensively with one another. Each hemisphere is responsible for processing information in a different way.

Eric R. Kandel in **the Disordered Mind: What Unusual Brains Tell Us about ourselves (2018),** writes *"Studies show that the left and right hemispheres of the brain deal with different aspects of mental functions and that the two hemispheres inhibit each other. Specifically, damage to the left hemisphere can free up the creative capabilities of the right hemisphere. More generally, when one neural circuit in the brain is turned off, another circuit, which was inhibited by the inactivated circuit, may turn on."*

During fetal development, genes determine where the neurons travel in the brain and their specialization. In addition to the need for neurons (brain cells) to migrate to all areas of the brain, we also need neuron circuits (wiring) to connect to various areas in the brain.

The neuron cells have extensions (axons) that allow communication to flow from cell to cell. Each axon (like an electrical cord) becomes covered in a white substance, called a myelin sheath, providing insulation and allowing the messages to convey at a faster speed. It can be thought of as covering on lamp wires. If the covering is incomplete, the electrical message may be disrupted and the light may blink or not come on at all.

If anything affects the formation of the myelin, then the quality of the signals will be changed. In multiple sclerosis (MS) scar tissue (sclerosis) forms when the myelin is destroyed. The brain is then unable to send and receive messages to the affected areas. The symptoms observed will depend on which nerves are affected and the severity of the damage.

Basilis Zikopoulos, Ph.D., and Helen Barbas*, Ph.D., from Boston University have examined postmortem brain tissue from individuals with and without autism. They found axons from autism brain tissue traveling to distant brain areas have less myelin (which would disrupt the quality of the signal going through the axon). In addition to problems with the covering (myelin) on these axons, children with autism also have problems with lack of connections to various areas of the brain.

In 2005, Eric Courchesne and Karen Pierce published *"Why the frontal cortex might be talking only to itself: local over-connectivity and long-distance disconnection."* Numerous studies now confirm that children with autism lack sufficient long-distance connections to process incoming information with meaning.

Split-brain Patients

Another approach to understanding how altered brain structure and function affect behavior is to study patients who may have these alterations as a result of surgery or trauma. Scientists have studied patients who have had this cable (corpus callosum) surgically cut that separates the two brain hemispheres, to stop epileptic seizures. They are called split-brain patients. These studies had startling results.

After the surgery, the patients report everything is fine and they don't notice any differences. But some creative scientists found ways of testing these patients that revealed the different functions of the left and right hemispheres and the importance of the connections between them. When the two hemispheres are connected, they work together, but when they are disconnected, they work separately creating strange results.

The studies revealed that the left hemisphere is the interpreter of input; it gives meaning to what we see. It is what enables us to see pictures in the clouds. It creates unity to the details; it sees the whole. The right hemisphere focuses on details. It would be impossible to remember all the details from day to day events, so the left hemisphere is designed to interpret cause and effect and attach meanings to create a general idea or gist.

In split-brain patients, the right hemisphere can read words and relate words to pictures, but it is the left hemisphere that can put the words together into a concept – creating meaning. The right hemisphere is literal – it can identify a dozen roses - but the left hemisphere is the interpreter and can add romance and emotion to the dozen roses. The brain connections are essential to processing concepts or main ideas.

This brain deficit of lack of long-distance connections in the brain is reflected in the symptoms of children with autism, who attend to details, but have difficulties processing meaning to understand main ideas. Temple Grandin writes in **The Way I See It** (2008) *"Many children and people with autism are not able to take all the facts they know and link them together to form concepts."*

Researchers at the University of Utah led by neurologist Dr. Jeffery Anderson and principal investigator, Dr. Janet Lainhart, used diffusion tensor (MRI) brain imaging to identify areas where the left and right hemispheres of the brains of people with autism do not communicate with one another. Without these long-distance connections, children with autism can process details in the right hemisphere, but fail to connect details with the main concept or big picture.

We automatically interpret meaning to details (social cues) in the environment and it is difficult to understand someone who cannot do this. David was a teenager working in a restaurant, clearing dishes from the tables. A man returned to his table from the restroom to find David had removed the dishes, when the man was not finished eating. To make a judgment of whether patrons are finished eating, we automatically interpret social situations from observed clues in the environment. The right brain attends to the details and the left brain adds meaning to the details. This enables us to make a plan of action. We do this so naturally, we take it for granted.

Let me describe some other behaviors seen in children with autism that reflect the focus on details and inability to process the main idea. When David was in preschool, he was sitting at the table with other children to have a snack. Suddenly, he stood up and started screaming. The crackers were star-shaped and he had only experienced crackers in a round shape. He could not observe and imitate his classmates, and his brain was unable to create a general concept of cracker that included multiple shapes, colors and tastes. His brain processed only one detail (right brain) and failed to process details into a general concept (left brain interpreter). Without the proper connections between the right and left hemisphere, you cannot process information adequately.

David loved alphabet letters, so I gave him the alphabet where each letter was on individual tiles. One day, he started throwing some of the tiles across the room. Upon closer inspection, I noticed that the tiles he threw had a letter with a line under it to distinguish the M from the W. From David's perspective, the letters were incorrect because of the line underneath them and from my perspective the line served a meaningful purpose. Behavior needs to be understood from the child's point of view. I helped him throw the tiles into the trashcan (a more appropriate behavior), because they didn't work for him.

One day, David was sitting at the table doing a craft with a "glue stic." He suddenly left the table. I patiently waited and watched. He found a pencil and came back to add a (K) to correct the spelling to "stic(K)" because he thought it was misspelled.

There are numerous behaviors (or symptoms) in autism that reflect this brain abnormality where the child focuses on details, such as play, exploratory behaviors and language development.

Play Behaviors

Pretend play is imitating behavior the child has observed in others. Children don't learn to imitate, but learn by imitating. Jean Piaget postulated a developmental theory that children learn to imitate in their second year of life because they start pretend play. Science now demonstrates that newborns have the ability to learn by imitating adults. Therefore, they don't have to learn how to imitate.

Children with autism do not have imitation or pretend play. The play is described as stereotyped, repetitive and rigid. It reflects how the child thinks based on how his brain works. The young child plays by himself, usually in a repetitive way, such as lining up letters in a pattern across the floor or stacking blocks and knocking them down. He may be preoccupied with parts of objects, such as spinning the wheels of a toy car or spinning the eyes of a toy monkey, but fail to appreciate the toy as symbolic of the family vehicle or an animal.

Typical children develop symbolic play by the third year of life. This is the ability to have a toy become symbolic or representative of something in real life. A stick can be a gun or a sword. A baby doll represents a real baby and a toy car represents the family car. This requires the ability to identify the object (toy) and interpret various meanings to the object.

Sometimes educators attempt to teach a child with autism pretend play, but if the child can't associate the meaning or social intent of the behavior, they are simply learning a routine. That is why children with autism have to be taught skills in real-life situations, because it incorporates meaning with the behaviors.

Exploratory Behavior

The behavior of children with autism reflects how their brains attend to details, but fails to connect meaning to the details. When you attend to the parts, the whole disappears; and when you attend to the whole, the parts disappear. When the child focuses only on a detail, it results in a lack of exploratory behavior.

When David was eight years old, I tried to prepare him for a neighborhood Easter egg hunt. I hid the eggs and then gave him a basket to find the eggs and fill the basket. After repeating the process three times, I realized he was looking at the same spots where I had hidden the eggs the first time. Even when the eggs were positioned in an open area, he failed to see them. He only attended to one detail of the "hunt" – the location of the eggs from the first experience. Because his brain was unable to connect to the meaning of the hunt as exploratory, he was unable to participate.

Karen Pierce and Eric Courchesne from UCLA, San Diego have studied the lack of exploratory behavior in children with autism. They connected the symptoms of restricted range of interests and stereotyped behaviors in children with autism with a structural abnormality in the cerebellum of the brain. Specifically, they identified hypoplasia – a failure of a part to grow or develop – in areas of the cerebellum. It was a surprise to researchers to find abnormalities in autism in this part of the brain, because it is considered our primitive brain.

In their 2001 article **"Evidence for a Cerebellar Role in Reduced Exploration and Stereotyped Behavior in Autism,"** Pierce and Courchesne concluded that *"Young autistic and normal children react in distinctly different ways when presented with an opportunity to explore and learn."* Normal children in the study spent 88% of their time in exploratory behavior and autistic children only spent 42% of their time in active exploratory behavior. In addition, the autistic children spent 27% of their time in *"repetitive activities, such as hand flapping, eye fluttering, or spinning objects, a type of behavior not seen in normal children."*

Parents and teachers are often baffled when the child does not have typical exploratory play behaviors. Most people are familiar with the Wheel of Fortune game show where one guesses letters until enough letters are revealed to enable one to guess the phrase and this solves the puzzle. David had a Wheel of Fortune hand-held game where one person could enter a puzzle for another person to solve. David wanted to watch me enter the puzzle and then he would "solve" the puzzle. From my perspective, the puzzle had been solved because he knew what it was by watching me enter it. But he had a different perspective of simply enjoying putting the letters into the proper spaces. Without an understanding of his different perspective, we could have had a conflict with me trying to force him to do the puzzle my way.

Pierce and Courchesne also reported that animal studies have linked abnormal structure and function of parts of the cerebellum with deficits in exploratory behaviors. I was surprised that the behaviors described in the animal research were behaviors I have observed in my own child with autism. For example, one study noted the tendency to circle the periphery of a novel environment. When David was a toddler, we took him to visit his grandparents. He would walk around the boundary of the property. At our home, David would take the same route out the back door to the swing and the same route back into the house – never taking a different route.

Social Interaction and Emotion related to Brain Function

When babies can identify faces and emotions in faces, they begin to socially interact with their caretakers. The typical newborn's brain processes nonverbal input through eye contact, facial expressions and tones of voice.

During the first year of life, both mother and baby often focus on the same object (called joint referencing) and this is a shared form of communication. This innate understanding is important for survival. Human babies are born helpless. They attend to faces and can imitate human faces almost immediately. They are wired for survival. It is important that they learn to identify emotions in faces to determine whom to trust. This interaction between mother and child is the beginning of the development of empathy and socialization.

A typical toddler has an invisible rubber band attached to the mother. The child may toddle a short distance away, but will maintain a nonverbal connection and soon returns to the mother. The lack of observation and imitation in children with autism disrupts the normal development of this connection between mother and child. A child with autism lacks the rubber band attachment to the mother and can get into dangerous situations. Unfortunately, there have been children with autism lost in the swamps, the mountains and killed by oncoming trains. You can call them and they do not respond.

When we observe faces, we typically simulate the emotional expression of the face we see. To understand emotion in others, we need to connect the facial expression with our own understanding of emotions. The mirror neuron network enables us to interpret and interact with others and our environment. Those who have a high degree of empathy have mirror neurons that react strongly to the actions of others. This system enables us to understand the actions and intentions of others.

When we go to the movies, we interpret the emotions of the actors because our mirror neurons enable us to "feel" the emotion they are feeling. If it is a scary movie, we feel fear; if it is romantic, we feel love; if it is a comedy, we feel humor and happiness. Without the brain structures and connections that enable us to interpret the facial expressions and distinguish one face from another, we would not be able to identify emotions and develop empathy for another person. We would have difficulty distinguishing the characters in a movie from one scene to another, understand the emotional displays, or follow the plot.

The ability to understand emotions also depends on long-distance connections in the brain to identify the emotion and connect it with the meaning of the emotion. For example, if I observe someone crying after falling, I associate the meaning (pain) with the behavior (crying). If I observe someone crying who is receiving an award, I associate meaning (happiness) with the behavior (crying). Notice this involves flexibility in thinking where one can associate different meanings for the same behavior.

Most people tend to attribute feelings, intentions and motivations to inanimate objects as well as people. Children often do this with a doll. Remember Tom Hanks with the volleyball in the movie, *"Cast Away"*? Jeff Dunham, a ventriloquist, gets the audience to empathize with his puppets. We do this so automatically that it is hard to imagine someone who is unable to do it.

Children with autism baffle us when they don't respond or express emotions in a manner we expect. Educators often try to teach identification and imitation of emotions. I was trying to teach my son to identify emotions in faces. I showed him pictures and I imitated the emotions. Finally, my son said, *"eyes open, happy; eyes closed, sad."* I reviewed the cards and discovered he was correct. He connected one detail of the face with the emotions of happiness and sadness. The brain would normally process the whole face and connect it to the emotions seen in the face. Typical babies do this without being taught, but when a child has a mirror neuron deficit and does not learn by observation and imitation, they focus on details and fail to process more meaning to what they see.

Children with autism often fail to express emotions during what should be highly emotional situations. For example, when my mother-in-law was dying of cancer, we were living in Lincoln, Nebraska and we went to North Carolina to stay with her, so I could provide nursing care in the home. One day, David said *"Is Nanny going to die so I can go to summer camp?"* He was not purposely being insensitive and he had a good relationship with his grandmother, but he had a greater need to know what to expect and he does not understand and express emotions in the typical manner. Empathy is a brain function and varies among individuals. Those who lack empathy for others, we often perceive as inconsiderate or obtuse.

Patients who have brain damage enable us to understand how someone cannot process emotions. Dr. Restak (**The Modular Brain** 1994) writes: *"The person with right brain damage inhabits a world where he can* *feel and experience the mind's major emotions but he cannot verbally express them or recognize and appropriately respond to emotions in others."* Temple Grandin writes in **Thinking in Pictures** (1995) *"My emotions are simpler than those of most people. I only understand simple emotions, such as fear, anger, happiness, and sadness. I don't know what complex emotion in a human relationship is."* Complex emotions (such as arrogance, pride, and jealousy) require long distance connections with the frontal lobes for processing.

Children with autism have great difficulties associating meaning with what they see, such as body gestures, including the language of the eyes. We typically interpret various meanings to our expressions with eyes, such as: 1) demonstrate you are listening to someone; 2) show anger, boredom, or flirtation; and 3) to indicate you want to say something. We need to understand that brain function determines how one thinks and learns. Children with autism do not automatically process meaning with what they see and hear, making social interaction extremely difficult.

Unstructured social situations are uncomfortable for people with autism, because their brains are different, and they do not process emotions in the typical manner. They cannot understand the unwritten rules of social behavior that rely to a great degree on gestures. They prefer structured situations where they know what to expect and what behaviors are required in the situation.

Temple Grandin tells us that autistics often associate emotions (positive and negative) with a particular place, more than a person. For example, we had an accident with a travel trailer, where we ran off the road and into the trees. I tried to talk with David to explain we had an accident and he remained calm the entire time. No one was hurt, so the policeman took us to get a rental car, so we could drive home. The next weekend, we returned to the site of the accident, and when we stopped the car, David started kicking and screaming. Since he had been calm during the accident itself, I was surprised by this reaction, but remembered Temple Grandin's information. David expressed a fear reaction to a place or location. He associated one detail (location) with the accident and was unable to create and access any other memory to the accident. When I told him we were safe, but just stopping to look for trailer parts in the ditch, he calmed. We cannot interpret autistic behaviors from a typical point of view.

Lack of Facial Recognition

With a deficit in mirror neuron function resulting in the lack of observation and imitation, we would expect people with autism to have difficulties with face identification and interpreting emotions in faces, because when they look at faces, it has no meaning for them. Temple Grandin writes, *"I often get into embarrassing situations because I do not remember faces unless I have seen the people many times or they have a very distinct facial feature, such as a big beard, thick glasses or a strange haircut."* When my son, David, was little, he would often refer to someone based on one feature, such as the nose, glasses or long dark hair.

The identification of faces occurs in the right hemisphere (right temporal lobe structure – the fusiform gyrus). One study by Karen Pierce and colleagues at the University of California demonstrated that <u>all</u> autistic individuals studied had reduced activation in this area and could not identify faces. The inability to recognize faces limits social interactions and needs to be recognized and supported.

I was unaware that David did not recognize faces until he was eleven years old. One day, I was talking with a neighbor, named Bill, and David did not greet him. I said to David, *"Say hello to Bill."* David responded, *"Which Bill?"* We had two "Bills" in our neighborhood and this one is over six feet tall! This was my first indication that David was unable to recognize faces.

We can learn from patients who have brain deficits that reflect various dysfunctions, such as face blindness. A patient suffered a stroke and when he awakened, he could not recognize faces, including his own. He recognized his wife by the sound of her voice. Although he could see clearly, the stroke damaged the brain in the area of facial recognition. When this occurs, it is a neurological deficit that cannot be cured.

What would happen if a patient (from stroke or trauma) could not connect his mother's face with the emotion associated with the face? When the patient looks at his mother's face, he will fail to feel the emotion usually associated with her face, so he concludes that she is an imposter. This "delusion" is called Capgras syndrome. In years past, we would probably consider the patient delusional and mentally ill. It is only through the understanding of brain function that we are able to appreciate the various behaviors that can result from brain deficits.

Face blindness is a brain deficit that cannot be fixed by education and must be accommodated. As long as educators are not taught about the neurological impairments of autistic children, they will continue to try to teach to deficits.

Genes determine Brain Connections

Our learning abilities depend on the structure and function of the brain and that depends mainly on our genes. During pregnancy, genes direct the movements of cells that build the structure and function of the brain. What causes abnormal brain development? How do brains create the connections to various areas in order to combine meaning with details? During this time of prenatal development -- particularly the 12th to the 25th week -- the brain cells in DNA can be altered or killed by genetic mutations or environmental insults, such as x-rays, toxins, drugs and alcohol, resulting in devastating conditions such as epilepsy, mental retardation, fetal alcohol syndrome and autism. These environmental insults can result in nerve cells not reaching some areas of the brain. Without proper development of nerve cells, normal learning cannot occur. Dr. Margaret Bauman, a pediatric neurologist with the Autism Research Foundation in Boston, states autism results from a lack of normal brain cell growth while the mother is pregnant.

In 2001, scientists discovered one gene that was altered during gestation that disrupted the brain's normal structure and function resulting in a serious speech and language disorder in some members of a family. Although we have two copies of every gene, a mutation in just one gene can have devastating effects on brain development. Researchers (Simone, Fisher, Anthony Monaco and colleagues) from the University of Oxford in England discovered the FOXP2 gene when they studied 15 members of a family with speech and language difficulties who inherited this problem. Another researcher – Jane Hurst – facilitated this identification when she found a British boy, unrelated to this family, who had an almost identical language deficit.

This gene produces a protein that plays an important role in brain development including the connections between brain cells. The scientists were surprised that such a small change in one gene could have such devastating results. One of the scientists (Monaco) reported that this gene is not responsible for *"less severe language deficits that affect approximately 4 percent of schoolchildren."* Scientists are now exploring the possibility of a mutation of FOXP2 being associated with autism but this is only one gene and there are numerous – as yet unidentified – genes associated with autism.

There are numerous possible gene deficiencies that cause the brain deficits in autism and this would account for some of the variations in behaviors observed. At this point, we have not been able to identify all the genes that are involved in autism, so there is no cure. It is unfair to parents for anyone to suggest or claim that they know how to cure autism. Although a search for a cure may be an appropriate goal, it is not likely in the near future. In the meantime, we need to find ways to help individuals with autism adapt to the world.

Genes determine the proper development of the brain and long-distance connections, but these connections are strengthened and some connections eliminated during childhood. As we learn and strengthen connections in the brain, we also have certain times – early childhood and adolescence – when some connections are pruned or eliminated. This is like pruning a tree – cutting off some of the branches, so the nutrients go to strengthen the remaining branches.

Jennifer Levitt and Xua Hua, UCLA researchers, reported in <u>Science Daily</u> that delays in autistic brain development continue into adolescence, with autistic brains growing much slower and unused cells not properly pruned away. Hue reported, *"...this creates unusual brain circuits with cells that are overly connected to their close neighbors and under-connected to important cells further away, making it difficult for the brain to process information in a normal way."*

Brain science also reveals that there is a link between some disorders that appear to be unrelated. For example, Eric R. Kandel in **The Disordered Mind: What Unusual Brains tell us about ourselves (2018)** writes: *"both autism and schizophrenia involve synaptic pruning, the removal of excess dendrites on neurons. In autism, not enough dendrites are pruned, whereas in schizophrenia too many are."* Also, *"Some of the same genes that create a risk for schizophrenia also create a risk for autism spectrum disorders."*

Language and Brain Function

The lack of long-distance connections in the brain will impact the autistic child's development of language. Parents are often most concerned about the lack of language in their children with autism. We often mistakenly think if the child can speak, then he can learn language. Many of us were taught a theory that babies are born as blank slates and we teach them everything that they know, including language. This is the basis of teaching language with behaviorism (ABA). But science has discovered that this is wrong. Our brains come prewired to learn language – if they are wired properly.

Much of science is discovered by accident and scientists were stunned to discover a newly created language from the brains of young children in Nicaragua. It was a unique situation that could not be created by a science experiment.

Sara Kennedy wrote an article in 2014, called ***"Children in Nicaragua Teach Scientists about Language."*** Deafness in Nicaragua was a stigma, so deaf children had little contact with each other and illiteracy was common. When the first schools opened for deaf children in 1981, the children began to communicate with each other. Although no one actually taught them to sign, the children started with simple pantomime and signs creating a system of gestures to communicate with one another. The children created Nicaraguan Sign Language (NSL) that followed the basic rules common to all languages (both spoken and signed), even though they were not taught these rules. This demonstrated that some language traits are not passed on by culture, but come from how the human brain processes information.

Typical children in different cultural settings all learn to point with their index finger by 14 months of age to communicate with caretakers. They also tend to look where another person is looking. They aren't taught to do this, but their brains are wired to learn this way, so they do it automatically.

Michael Gazzaniga in **Who's in Charge?** (2011) wrote *"babies everywhere know the same stuff at the same age no matter what they have been exposed to."* He wrote that babies possessed the following knowledge even without language: 1) Objects are permanent and do not disappear when blocked from view; 2) Objects are solid and do not break apart when tugged and do not pass through other objects; 3) Objects keep the same shape when they disappear and reemerge; and 4) Objects move in a continuous path. Rather than born blank-slates, babies have brains designed to learn even before learning language.

Nora Schultz wrote an article in New Scientist (2011) called *"Baby apes' arm waving hints at origins of language."* She writes *"The emerging gesture theory of language evolution has it that our ancestors' linguistic abilities may have begun with their hands rather than their vocal cords."* Studies of apes show that they develop a complex repertoire of gestures during the first two years of life.

In order for gestures to be effective, the young ape must be aware of the meaning of the gestures and that another ape must be paying attention, if they want to get their message across. The young apes do, in fact, get the attention of another ape – by pokes and gestures – before communicating. Typical children, by the second year of life, understand that they need to get the attention of another person in order for the communication to be effective. The child usually points and looks at the mother, to see if she is watching. Sometimes, the child will pull the mother's arm to get her attention.

Gestures require interpreting social meaning.

Gestures may be the basis of learning language, but many children with autism lack an understanding of the social meaning of gestures. A child may be able to interpret sounds into language and connect meanings with words, but fail to process meaning to gestures. If the child is concentrating on interpretation of speech, he is ignoring the gestures and failing to process social aspects of speech. Since gestures may be indicative of the origins of speech and children with autism fail to process gestures properly, this helps explain the social communication problems with autism.

Some children with autism fail to understand that communication occurs with other human beings. For example, we had taught David to order his flavor of ice cream in an ice cream store. One day, he walked up to the counter and announced *"David wants vanilla,"* but the clerk was in the back room talking on the telephone. We don't teach typical children that they have to speak to another person in order to communicate, because we assume everyone knows that. When we recognize the child with autism does not understand the purpose of speech as a form of communication with another human being, then his behavior begins to make sense.

David was <u>nine</u> years old and I heard him making a request in a room by himself. The behavior clearly indicates he does not understand he has to speak to a human being! We sometimes interpret this as a failure to take the perspective of another person, but the deficit is more basic than that. We don't teach children that they need to share thoughts and ideas with another person, because their brains process this intuitively. But children with autism do not understand the purpose of communication and this is reflected in their behaviors.

David went through a period where he would respond to anyone asking a question, even if it was not directed toward him. We were standing in a grocery line and the clerk was talking to the customer in front of us. It was a yes/no question, and David answered it. He had difficulty determining when someone was speaking to him. This was probably due to the mirror neuron deficit resulting in lack of observation and discerning meaning to what he sees and hears.

Charles Hart in his book, **Without Reason**, noted his son, Ted, was reading a book and he asked the question, *"What is this?"* He failed to understand that he had to show the book to his father in order to properly communicate with him. We don't normally teach children communicative intent, because our brains are designed to do this.

We need to be cognizant of this deficit in order to help the child with autism adapt to the world. Basic communicative behaviors, such as facing those you are trying to communicate with, are missing in autism. When David was doing gymnastics, he was to face the judge and salute to indicate he was ready to start his routine. He had to be specifically taught these behaviors.

On another occasion, he was receiving an award on stage and he did not face the audience, so he had to be turned around. When ordering in a restaurant, he would look at the menu and speak in a low voice. We had to teach him to turn his face toward the person taking his order and speak loud enough for the server to hear. Please note that the instructions were not to *"make eye contact,"* because that had no meaning for him and could be distracting.

Details and Language

The ability to combine words to create greater meaning requires long distance connections between the two hemispheres in the brain. The split-brain patients demonstrate this difficulty, because they can identify "water" and "pail" (right hemisphere), but will fail to put "water into a pail" (left hemisphere). They can identify roses, but fail to add more meaning – such as love and romance.

Children with autism have deficient long-distance connections between the two hemispheres and demonstrate deficits similar to split-brain patients. They can connect a label or meaning to one word, but without long-distance connections to the left hemisphere, they will fail to interpret multiple meanings to a word or the meaning of a sentence as different from the meaning of a word or two within a sentence. In addition, changing the order of the words in a sentence can change the meaning of the sentence, and this makes learning language very difficult for children with autism.

Dr. Restak writes (**The Modular Brain**. 1994) about a patient who *"lost the ability to extract meaning from a sentence despite a retained ability to understand the meaning of each of the words in isolation."* This is a patient who had the ability prior to a brain trauma and then lost that ability. Children with autism may not have the ability to begin with and we need to consider this when we are trying to teach language.

Some children with autism can read (decode words), but have difficulties understanding the meaning of what they read. The decoding of words occurs in one area of the brain and the meaning is processed in other areas. It requires brain connections between all these areas.

When teaching reading comprehension to David, it had to be related to something he was doing, so it had meaning for him. He could not relate to what someone else was doing. He played computer games, so he read game strategies and this made sense to him. With cooking, he reads each step of the recipe before he does it. Comprehension increases when it is associated with what the child is doing.

A patient who has a stroke in the left hemisphere in the speech area may be able to understand some language and be able to speak, but have difficulty processing complex speech. For example, the patient may be able to

125

identify an antelope and a lion, but fail to process the sentence: *"The antelope was killed by the lion."* Which animal died? The patient may only process antelope –killed – lion.

Inability to process complex speech means the child with autism will have great difficulty attaching meaning to jokes, concepts, idioms, metaphors and so on. People with right frontal lobe damage also fail to understand jokes and they prefer slapstick humor. In studies of adults with frontal lobe damage, the patient is given several options and asked to choose an appropriate ending to a joke, but they can't do it. The understanding of jokes requires the ability to apply meaning to the situation and then recognize a shift in meaning.

Secrets Revealed

The lack of observation and imitation was identified over two hundred years ago, and science has finally discovered the brain abnormalities that result in these symptoms. The discovery of mirror neurons shows these cells enable us to observe and imitate, to attach meaning to what we observe and to distinguish between our own movements and the movements of others.

Children with autism lack observation and imitation and this is confirmed by a variety of approaches in brain science: 1) Motor mirror neurons are involved in the ability to observe and imitate; 2) Structural abnormality in the cerebellum resulting in lack of pretend play that requires observation and imitation; 3) Lack of facial recognition required for observing and imitating facial expressions (emotion); and, 4) lack of ability to process gestures and emotions in others resulting in social deficits.

Karen Pierce and Eric Courchesne showed a structural abnormality in the cerebellum of the brain, so children with autism have difficulties with pretend play and exploratory play, resulting in repetitive and rigid play behaviors. Animal studies also confirm this. Drs. Itard and Seguin revealed over 200 years ago, that the children they taught failed to play with typical toys and had to learn skills in the environment where it would be used.

Brain research has demonstrated: 1) Children with autism have gene mutations that result in the lack of long distance connections. Genes determine where the neurons travel and their specialization; 2) The corpus callosum connection between the two hemispheres is smaller in people with autism; 3) The axons (extensions of brain cells) traveling to distant brain areas have less myelin (insulation), which would disrupt the quality of the signal; 4) There are delays in brain development in children with autism, with autistic brains growing much slower and unused cells not properly pruned away; and 5) Studies on split-brain patients, who have the long-distance connections severed, demonstrate that the two hemispheres process information differently. The right brain processes details and the left brain is the interpreter and connects details to create the main idea or general concept.

In the last chapter, we discovered that children with autism may feel sensations, but not attach meaning to the sensation. They may see objects, but not know what they are seeing, because they are unable to connect the meaning of the object. Perceptions of our sensations require long-distance connections in the brain, and brain science demonstrates the lack of long-distance connections in autism.

Eric R. Kandel writes in **The Disordered Mind: What Unusual Brains Tell Us about Ourselves,** that our incoming sensations are processed for meaning *"by making unconscious perceptual information in wide areas of the cerebral cortex, especially the prefrontal cortex, the part of the brain responsible for integrating perception, memory, and cognition"*. We know children with autism have deficient long-distance connections to the prefrontal cortex that enable one to process meaning to sensations including associating it with past experiences.

This helps us understand behaviors of young children with autism. For example, why would a young child when given a snack including a star shaped cracker, suddenly start screaming? His brain fails to connect to the prefrontal cortex to process meaning. He needs memories to connect the new shape of the cracker with the round shape he is familiar with to enable him to decide on a response. Being unable to process meaning of this strange object, he screams until someone removes it from the table. His brain does not enable him to make a plan of action to get rid of the offending cracker.

What are some of the symptoms that result from the lack of long-distance connections? Without the proper long-distance connections between the hemispheres, children with autism will attend to details, but fail to develop general concepts in memory. Examples include: 1) Child may understand the meaning of individual words in a sentence, but fail to comprehend the meaning of the sentence; 2) Child fails to understand the meaning or intent of language to communicate with another person; 3) Child may relate words to pictures, but fail to put the words together into an interpretation; 4) Child may identify a trash can in one environment because of a symbol (detail), but fail to identify trash cans in general (concept); and. 5) Lack of generalization results from focus on details and lack of concepts (memories) to plan behaviors in other environments or situations.

We have reviewed brain research from a variety of perspectives – normal development, single cell, genetics, brain imaging, post-mortem studies, neurological problems and psychological testing on split-brain patients. Yet, it all confirms the core brain deficits in autism are lack of observation and imitation from a mirror neuron system deficit and lack of long-distance connections resulting in attention to details, but failure to process details into greater meanings, main ideas, or concepts.

Professionals often make the mistake of teaching to the deficits identified in the psychiatric diagnostic criteria. For example, Dr. Lovaas (ABA) tried to teach imitation, proper toy play and interaction with peers. A recent (2015) article in the Journal of Autism and Developmental Disorders by Laura Schreibman, Geraldine Dawson, and colleagues stated that teaching observation and imitation would help children with autism learn. This reflects adherence to old environmental theories that everything can be taught. Brain science now reveals that newborns are born with brain structure and function that enable them to observe and imitate immediately. When the structure and function of the brain is different, the child will learn differently.

You would not try to teach a blind child to see, or teach to the deficit of a neurologically impaired patient, so it doesn't make any sense to teach to the deficits of a child with autism, who has a neurological impairment. Temple Grandin wrote that one of her teachers of math told her to "just listen" rather than try to write everything down. But she could not remember the sequence of steps. The teacher failed to recognize that people have learning differences. The knowledge of brain functions in autism should be the basis for teaching strategies.

We all have slightly different brains, because we have been exposed to different experiences. Genetics has shown us how genes dictate the organization of the brain and how changes in genes influence disorders. Brain imaging could be a powerful diagnostic tool for brain disorders and planning education and treatment.

The next chapter discusses memory and learning in autism.

Chapter 8

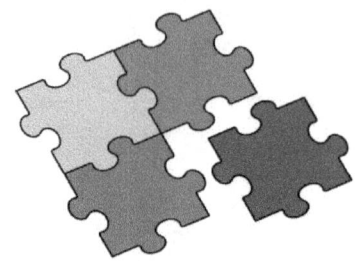

Memory and Learning

"If a child can't learn the way we teach, maybe we should teach the way they learn." Ignacio Estrada

Learning is the main activity of the brain and memory is the result of the learning process. Learning is the creation of memories resulting from our experiences. Learning also relies on the ability to retrieve these memories to allow us to talk about the past. When we retrieve memories, it enables us to generalize to future experiences. If we don't have memory then we can't remember the past or imagine the future. We are stuck in the present.

Memory is related to sensation and perceptions. If you fail to process the meaning of sensations, then you fail to create meaning – memory and meaning go together.

When we think of memory, we usually think of associative memory and this is a vital component of our everyday lives. It enables us to store information about what we have done in the past and retrieve it at another time. A memory does not exist in the brain as a unit. For example, when we encounter a cat, our brains process the details of what we see, hear, feel, and smell in locations all over the brain, and then the prefrontal cortex creates meaning to the input, but it occurs so rapidly and all comes together, so we perceive it as a unit. In other words, our knowledge of a concept (Memory) involves the linkage in the brain of various sensations and interpretations of those sensations.

A greater understanding of brain function enables us to consider how children with autism may perceive the world in a different manner than most of us do, because we have more complete brain wiring.

Associational Learning

Our associational learning results from how the brain typically functions. Every time a typical child goes into a store, she observes and imitates. A young child may push one of the mini carts, so she can imitate Mom. She may point (or grab) something she likes off the shelf. She learns and stores these experiences of her trips to the grocery store in associative memory. When she returns to the store, she retrieves her memories and adds more details to the general concept of shopping in the store.

When we look at something, the brain interprets the incoming sensations of what we see, hear, feel and touch with meaning (social intent) of our experiences. For example, the smell of fish may start a recall of being at the beach. Associational links enable the brain to connect the smell of fish with the sound of waves crashing on the beach, the sound of seagulls, and the memories of a previous vacation. It is why the sound of a particular song may start the retrieval of a past experience.

The reconstructing of memories relies on these fragments of sensory information. Memories are not stored in one area of the brain because memory consists of a relational network of sensory information. This relational or associative structure of memory in the brain enables meaning to combine with the various aspects of memory: meaning and memory intertwine. When the typical child returns to the store another time, she retrieves some memory of her previous visit. This enables her to build knowledge of what behaviors are expected in every environment. When a person accesses memories of previous experiences in a similar environment, this enables her to manage new or novel situations.

When a child with autism goes into a grocery store, he is not creating meaning to what he sees, so he is not creating or storing associative memories. Because the child with autism thinks and learns differently, he may associate a single detail to a place or experience. This does not enable the child to learn what behaviors are needed in an environment and he is unable to deal with novel situations.

Eric R. Kandel explains in **The Disordered Mind: What Unusual brains Tell Us about Ourselves (2018)**, that *"Studies show that the left and right hemispheres of the brain deal with different aspects of mental functions and that the two hemispheres inhibit each other. Specifically, damage to the left hemisphere can free up the creative capabilities of the right hemisphere. More generally, when one neural circuit in the brain is turned off, another circuit, which was inhibited by the inactivated circuit, may turn on."* For example, in autism when the associational learning circuit is turned off, other circuits, such as rote memory, can become highly active that the child can use to learn. In the examples of behaviors that follow, we will see how the child with autism can have an inactive associational memory and then will use his rote memory in his attempt to understand the world.

How do we know that a child with autism is not storing associative memories of his experiences? Some of the behaviors that indicate this problem are: 1) Can't speak of the past 2) Difficulty generalizing experiences to other environments; 3) Difficulty imagining a skill and imitating it; and 4) Difficulty planning for the future.

Speaking about the Past

One needs to access memories in order to talk about what one has done in the past. If a child with autism cannot remember what they have done during the day then they cannot tell you about it. For example, if I told David (age 12), *"Tell Daddy what we did today,"* he would look confused and say, *"Did we go to the grocery store?"* Despite the fact he had speech and going to the grocery store was a weekly training environment, he could not remember and tell us about it. Learning requires building memories through observation and imitation and storing them, so we can connect the past to the present and the future – it is mental time travel.

What would it be like to lack associative memories? Studying patients who have memory problems due to brain damage enables us to better understand the memory deficits that can occur in autism. We know where in the brain associational memories are created. There is a patient, H.M., who had his temporal lobes on both sides of his brain surgically removed to stop seizures. He lost his ability to form new associational memories. He forgot the events of daily life shortly after they occurred. He could meet and carry on a conversation with someone and then forget what was said or whom he talked with. Every day was like a new beginning.

H.M. could remember events from his childhood and early adult life prior to the surgery, so his old memories were intact, but he could not create new memories. How could this be? Dr. Restak (**The Modular Brain**. 1994) wrote about another patient, R.B., who suffered brain damage during cardiac bypass surgery and his associational memory was impaired just like H.M. With R.B., it was discovered that he only had damage to the hippocampus (a specific area of the brain), leading to the conclusion that the hippocampus is essential to create associational memories and then the memories are stored in various other areas of the brain. Without proper brain function of the hippocampus, one cannot build associational memories.

The hippocampus is involved in creating associative memory, so any alteration in the structure of the hippocampus would affect this function. Brain science has demonstrated impaired structure of the hippocampus in children with autism. In April 2007, Dager and colleagues reported a study in the <u>American Journal of Neuroradiology</u> (AJNR) called, "Shape Mapping of the Hippocampus in Young Children with ASD." They reported Hippocampal shape measures distinguished children with autistic disorder (AD) from those with typical development (N=13)...and within the ASD sample (N=45), the shape alterations distinguished the more severely affected children (autistic disorder) from the less severely affected children (PDD-NOS). Hippocampal shape alterations in children with ASD were correlated with degree of mental retardation and performance tests of MTL (Medial Temporal Lobe) function. This demonstrates that the differences in functioning of children with autism spectrum disorder correlates with the severity of the brain defect.

Research on neurotransmitters (chemical messengers in the brain) also demonstrates functional problems in the hippocampus. Scientists at the NYU Langone Medical Center discovered the chemical oxytocin acts on the hippocampus to improve information processing by enabling neurons to separate important information from background noise. Chemicals such as oxytocin, dopamine and serotonin act as chemical messengers between brain cells by activating receptors on the cell or preventing the activation of receptors on the cell. The scientists theorize that autism is associated with a genetic alteration of the oxytocin receptor (OXTR) so the person gets lost in the details, while ignoring the big picture or gestalt. The proper functioning of the hippocampus is essential to developing associational memories and this can be a deficit in autism.

Associational learning depends on proper brain function. In the last chapter, I mentioned the FOXP2 gene related to a speech and language disorder. Since the identification of FOXP2 gene, other scientists, MIT's Ann Graybiel and Svante Paabo from the Max Planck Institute, have demonstrated that introducing the human version of this gene into mice speeds up their associational learning. The altered mice were able to associate previous learning with new experiences and incorporate this into their behavior. They respond quickly to various details in the environment. Implanting a human version of FOXP2 gene into mice is a far cry from implanting into a human, but it is an important step.

Generalization

Teachers often refer to children with autism as lacking generalization. The child fails to transfer (generalize) a skill from one environment to another setting. This happens because the child fails to observe and imitate in the environment, so he can create memories of behaviors needed in each environment. Let's look at some examples.

Many children with autism cannot cross the street independently. When we teach children to cross the street, we tell them to stop, look both ways for hazards (such as cars and bicycles) and then cross when it is safe to do so. While the child is young, parents often take the child's hand when crossing the street. Because she observes and imitates, the typical child will combine the sensory details with the main idea (meaning) of these experiences and then store the information in associative memory. When the child encounters a situation where they need to cross the street, she will retrieve parts of the associative memory to enable her to apply it to a novel situation. This is generalization.

Although the child with autism may have crossed the street with a parent on many occasions, he will only cross the street safely at the location where he is specifically taught details. He fails to combine details with previous experiences to combine memory and meaning. Since there is no associative memory to retrieve, he will not be able to cross the street at another location. Therefore, the child has to be taught the skill in various locations by teaching to the details. For example, some locations have crossing guards, some have electric light controls, some have markings on the pavement and some areas do not. The child may look both ways and still not understand what he is looking for, and proceed to cross the street in front of a car.

There can be challenges with behaviors generalizing in every environment. One day, after eating in a fast-food restaurant, David could not find the trashcan. Looking for differences in the situation, it became apparent we had been going to McDonald's where the trashcan had a symbol on it. This restaurant lacked the symbol. Rather than creating an associative memory of eating in restaurants, he will only remember one small detail and this does not enable generalization to other environments.

The extent of the lack of generalization depends on the severity of autism (the severity of the brain disorder). Here is an example of a child with more severe autism. As a teenager, David was on a gymnastics team and they were practicing their floor routines. Several boys performed their floor routines and then it was David's turn. The coach directed him to the starting corner. David stood there and he did not start his routine.

I was sitting with parents behind a glass wall. I held my breath as the coach looked puzzled. What could be his problem? How we perceive the problem will determine how we respond to it. Was it a social problem of failing to imitate his peers? Was it a language problem reflecting a lack of understanding? The coach directed David to another corner of the floor and he performed beautifully.

The coach realized that during the individual lessons, David had done the floor routine from only one corner, so he perceived the other corners as different. During the next individual lesson, David was taught to perform a floor routine from any of the four corners. If we don't understand how the child thinks and learns, we may interpret the behavior as willfully defiant or lacking motivation. Rather than blame the child, we must learn to view behavior from a brain perspective.

The lack of generalization is also demonstrated in the speech of children with autism. The child may learn a word, but apply it to only one thing. For example, I told David, a toddler, to *"Put the block on the table."* The coffee table was in front of him, but he ran out of the room and put the block on the dining table. He associated the word "table" with only one table.

Behaviors begin to make sense when we understand the brain function of people with autism.

Temple Grandin is higher functioning on the Autism spectrum, so I wondered how she created associative memory that enabled her to generalize to other environments. In **Thinking in Pictures**, she explains how she connects meanings to words and concepts. She describes associating meaning with actions. Words had no meaning until she could associate the word with a physical movement. For example, she learned the word "under'" by associating it with getting under the cafeteria tables at school. Meanings are associated with pictures that she is able to store in memory. If she encounters a cat, she can retrieve pictures of cats in her memory and add new details to the concept. Dr. Grandin's associative memory is filled with pictures and videos. She remembers many events of her past as videos and can retrieve them. She states *"Even though my memories of things are stored as individual specific memories, I am able to modify my mental images."*

Children with autism learn differently, so we have to teach differently. They must be taught behaviors in every environment including different details. If the child only identifies one table, then we have to specifically identify tables in various environments. We don't have to do this for typical children. The brain function in autism makes it difficult for them to learn behaviors in different environments, because they don't create associative memories that can be retrieved to help them learn.

Memory and Imitation

One has to access memories in order to imagine doing something and then imitating it. V.S. Ramachandran in **The Tell-Tale Brain** (2011) discusses a condition called "apraxia" that results in difficulties with imitation. Patients who have this disorder are known to have deficits in the area of the parietal lobe involved in the production, comprehension and imitation of skills. Dr. Ramachandran writes that these people have difficulty imitating gestures and do not know when they are doing it wrong.

He writes that some people are unable to imagine how to perform a skill in order to imitate it, but if you give them an object, they can demonstrate how to use it, because they do not have to rely on imagination (memory). My son, David, who is 31 years old, demonstrates this difficulty.

When asked to pretend he is combing his hair, he will pat his head. But when given a comb, he is able to properly comb his hair.

This helps explain why children with autism have great difficulties with pretend play and imitation, but can learn to use objects in real-life activities. Typical children learn through pretend play, because they can imagine an activity and imitate it.

Since we teach typical young children through pretend play, we attempt to teach children with autism to learn in the same manner, but it doesn't work. It is important that we teach children with autism skills and activities using objects in real-life situations. If you try to teach pretend play to a child with autism, he learns a routine, because he cannot build on associational memories of previous observations.

Planning and Sequencing Skills

People with autism have difficulties with planning and sequencing skills. Remembering is thinking back in time, planning is thinking forwards in time and sequencing is putting events together as they are organized in time. It is mental time travel that relies on associative memory.

These deficits are identified in patients who have brain damage in the frontal lobes of the brain. Dr. Restak in **The Modular Brain** (1994) wrote about a patient who had a tumor in the right frontal lobe of her brain removed. After the surgery, the patient reported no problem, but she had great difficulty with organizing, scheduling and completing tasks. Dr. Restak noted that she managed routine tasks, but lacked flexibility of thinking to manage novel situations. He writes: *"The affected person loses the ability to initiate a plan of action, stick with it and reach a goal. Moreover, no generally available methods so far have proven successful in assisting frontal lobe patients with their planning difficulties."* There is no evidence that any teaching methods can cure brain deficits, so we have to teach to the strengths and accommodate the deficits.

Mental time travel is an integral part of associative memory and relies on the right frontal lobe of the brain. Drs. Eric Courchesne and Karen Pierce from UCLA have reported early growth abnormalities in the frontal lobes of the brain in people with autism. Their research indicates that in autism the wiring in the brain is over-connected locally (in the prefrontal cortex) and disconnected to other parts of the brain. Dr. Gazzaniga also confirms this disorder. He writes in **Who's in Charge?** (2011) *"a lesion in the lateral frontal lobes produces deficits in sequencing behavior, leaving one unable to plan or multitask.*

Planning to prepare a meal requires sequencing behavior – remembering the order of the steps. Therefore, one would expect a child with autism to have difficulties getting organized to cook, because it requires imagining what tools and food items are needed and where they are located. To accommodate this difficulty, a list of what is needed on the recipe may help the child function independently. Despite the fact my son may have made a recipe many times, he still relies on the written instructions to keep the sequence in order. The difficulties with multitasking are revealed when the child can only prepare one recipe at a time. It would be impossible to follow the sequence of steps, if one was trying to prepare several recipes at one time.

Dr. Temple Grandin writes about these challenges. In **The Way I See It: A personal Look at Autism and Asperger's** (2008), she writes that it was difficult for her to plan for the future. She states *"I had to use door symbolism to symbolize that I was going on to the next step in my life. When you think visually, and you don't have very much stuff on the (mental) hard drive from previous experiences, you've got to have something to use as a visual map."* She indicates a lack of associative memories (stuff on the hard drive from previous experiences), so she relies on visual symbolism to combine meaning with an experience to help her plan for the future. This is an example of how a high functioning person with autism adapts to future experiences.

Fortunately, Dr. Grandin has allowed researchers to perform multiple brain images to help us understand how she can function higher than others with autism. The images have shown that she has more connections through the corpus callosum that connects the left and right hemispheres of the brain. By having more long- distance connections, Dr. Grandin is able to create meaning with pictures and access those pictures through memory. She also states (Grandin 2014) *"My brain's language circuit branches more than a normal brain's..."* We know that there are multiple gene mutations in autism and not every person will have the exact same mutations, so there can be a variety of symptoms in autism.

Rote Memory

Some children with autism are able to develop an incredible internal map of how to get from point A to point B. David as a toddler would suddenly scream while we were in the car, if he thought we were going to the mall and I took a different route. Children with autism are often quite good at games that involve learning maps or mazes. This is rote memory for facts and is functionally quite distinct from memory of the self across time (associational memory).

Rote learning is a different type of learning circuit in the brain, and is based on doing something over and over until it becomes automatic – you don't have to think about it to do it. Rote learning is usually associated with such activities as learning the alphabet or multiplication tables as well as tying shoes, typing, riding a bike, or playing a piano. But rote learning can be used to teach a child with autism life skills.

Children with autism have excellent rote learning as revealed when they repeat definitions from a dictionary, bus schedules, commercial jingles, songs or poems. The National Research Council (2001) wrote in **Educating Children with Autism** that *"The ability to learn material by rote may be less impaired than that involved in the manipulation of more symbolic materials."* One has to question why we continue to teach children with autism to learn like typical children.

Over 200 years ago, Seguin identified the strength in rote memory and difficulties with associational memory in idiots (autistics). He wrote that it was quite common for these children to have great memory for musical imitation, counting, and mechanics, but they can't remember what they ate for dinner, or answer a question except by repeating the final word of the question. He also noted that many well-meaning attendants will teach these children long pieces of poetry, or the names of presidents, but this information has little meaning or value for the child.

We can see evidence that rote memory is a learning strength in children with autism, because they will repeat phrases that they have heard – often from television commercials. The commercials are easier to remember because they are often associated with music. These memorized phrases may become the main essence of their communication.

In the last section of the book, I will show you how to teach children with autism through rote memory. Associational learning enables one to connect meaning to what one does, but rote learning does not incorporate meaning with the skill. For example, the child with autism may be taught to do laundry by rote, but fail to recognize that after a cycle in the dryer, wet clothes are not ready to be put away. This requires understanding the purpose of the dryer is to dry clothes: it is the social intent of the activity. They understand the routine, but often fail to process the meaning or social intent or main concepts, because of deficient brain function.

We discussed previously how patients with damage to the hippocampus were unable to form new associational memories. Interestingly, they retained their skills learned by rote memory, but did not remember that they knew how to do these things. If patient H.B. was told to sit down at the piano and play something, he would not remember that he knows how until he starts to play. Therefore, you would not see him initiate behaviors.

We know that many children with autism often fail to reveal their skills learned by rote or to initiate an activity that they know how to do. Charles Hart in **Without Reason** (1989) wrote about his autistic brother and his autistic son. He stated that he had asked his son's teacher to teach Ted to tie his shoes. Months passed and he had not heard if Ted had learned to tie his shoes. When he asked the teacher, she was surprised as she had taught him months previously. The parents were continuing to tie his shoes, because they did not know he could do it himself and he did not tell them or initiate the behavior.

Charles Hart reported that when he went to visit his brother (60 years old), who was living in an institution, he noticed that his toenails were extremely long and his shoes were too big for him in order to accommodate the long toenails. When he asked the staff, they responded that they tried to cut his nails, but he resisted. Charles Hart was upset, because his brother had been cutting his own toenails for 50 years! He simply handed him the clippers, and he cut his own nails.

Teachers often make this mistake of teaching a child with autism a skill that they already know how to do, because the child does not say, *"I can do it myself"*. Caretakers often assume a child doesn't know how to do something, because they don't communicate or initiate the behavior.

Because children with autism think and learn differently, we must teach in a different manner. We need to support the brain deficits and teach to the strengths of details, rote learning, and active hands-on experiences in multiple environments. We must find and use the child's sensory strength for teaching and avoid using language that can be incorporated into a learning routine, as this can prevent independence.

Secrets Revealed

Typically, the brain learns by processing incoming sensations combined with meaning to create associative memory. We have learned that children with autism lack long-distance connections to process meaning with the sensations, so this affects their ability to form associative memories. Impaired sensory processing also affects associational learning because the reconstructing of memories relies on fragments of sensory information.

I discussed the structure and function of the hippocampus is affected in autism, as well as the chemical oxytocin that acts on the hippocampus to improve information processing by enabling neurons (brain cells) to separate important information from background noise. They theorize a genetic alteration of the oxytocin receptor in autism. Therefore, we have scientists studying the brain from the perspective of chemical transmitters (oxytocin) and the structure of the hippocampus with both demonstrating deficits in associative memory.

Brain science gives us the basis for creating teaching strategies for children with autism based on their learning strengths (rote learning) and weaknesses (associative memory). There will be deficits in remembering, planning, and sequencing behaviors. Remembering is thinking back in time, planning is thinking forward in time, and sequencing is putting events together as they are organized in time. Without the ability to remember past experiences, the child with autism will be unable to speak about what he did during the day, generalize behaviors to other environments, imagine a skill and imitate it and plan for the future. We can accommodate these deficits by 1) using pictures of what the child has done to create a memory of past events; 2) organize materials for a task to assist the child with planning; and, 3) support sequencing difficulties with visuals and teaching to rote memory.

The differences need to be accommodated by teaching through the child's dominate sensory strength, and teaching to rote memory (doing the same thing over and over until it becomes automatic). The third section of the book will discuss how to teach, what to teach and why you are teaching it based on brain structure and function.

Section Three: Teaching Strategies for Autism

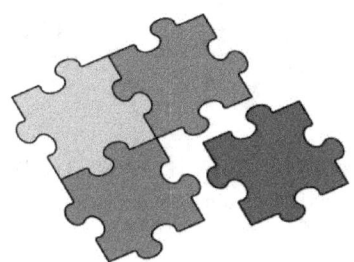

Chapter 9

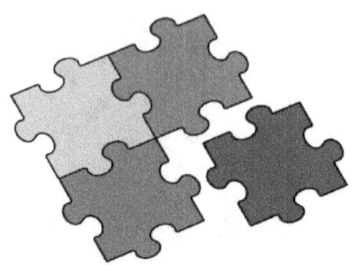

Learn Differently; Teach Differently

The single biggest problem in communication is the illusion that it has taken place.
George Bernard Shaw.

Dr. Temple Grandin has been telling us for decades that children with autism think and learn differently. Autism is a neurological disorder and brain science defines the strengths and differences in autism that can guide us toward developing more appropriate teaching strategies.

Abnormalities of sensation and perception affect our brain processing capabilities, and must be better understood when addressing the educational needs of children with autism. Sensations refer to sensing our environment through touch, taste, smell, sight and sound. Perception involves judgment and interpretation of the world, rather than a passive reaction to sensory input. It relies on brain function.

Learn Differently; Teach Differently

In **Thinking in Pictures** (1995), Temple Grandin writes: *"Because children with autism can see and hear then we assume they need to be taught through those senses and that is the way we teach typical children. But the child may learn better through a different sense."* When we describe behaviors based on sensory processing difficulties, they no longer seem bizarre and begin to make sense. Sensations and perceptions are based on how the brain works and it does not work the same in everyone. Temple Grandin has been telling us about sensory problems for decades, yet professionals continue to ignore these issues

Multiple sensations presented at the same time may cause circuit overloads and the child may shut down completely. Typical children enjoy environments with intense sensory input, but children with autism may become overwhelmed and exhibit aberrant behaviors. Whenever strange behaviors occur, one should reevaluate the teaching procedures and provide more support for the child. I provide numerous examples of how to respond to a child's strange behaviors in various situations.

We can provide many accommodations for the sensory and perceptual differences in autism, such as squeeze machines, soft fabric, quiet environments with reduced visual and auditory distractions, earphones in some environments to reduce auditory noise, a baseball cap that reduces visual distractions and opportunities to help the child understand and use objects that may initially frighten him.

In addition, we need to provide teaching strategies that rely on the child's sensory learning strengths. Children with autism may be unable to process information through two sensory inputs at the same time, such as auditory and visual (show and tell).

For example, they may respond to what they hear and ignore what they see. When David was young, I stood in front of the refrigerator holding two cartons of milk. I asked David to "Open the door." David ran to the front door of the house and opened the door. He responded to my words, but did not process meaning to seeing me stand in front of the refrigerator. This is the type of behavior that baffles parents and educators, but is explained by the lack of long-distance connections in the brain, that prevent the child from combing meaning with everything he hears and sees.

One time, I took David to the barber shop and when it was David's turn to get a haircut, the barber was standing behind the chair and said, *"Time for a haircut young man,"* as he tapped the chair with his hand. Of course, David sat in the empty chair where he sat the last time he had a haircut, but it was not the chair the barber was standing behind. We have to recognize that children with autism may often only process information through one sensory channel, so we need to use that channel more effectively.

Our verbal communication needs to be very specific to include social meaning from lack of observation. For example, David is 31 years old and I told him to look at what I put in the birdbath. I was standing by the kitchen window, pointing to the birdbath. He went to a different window and looked at the birdbath in the back of the house. We have two birdbaths and once again, he responded to my words and ignored my gestures. I confess to being a slow learner!! I should have told him to *"Look out this window at the bird bath and you can see the bird statue."*

Children with autism may be *"blind but can see."* Temple Grandin writes in **The Way I See It** (2008) *"Eye contact is still difficult for me in noisy rooms because it interferes with hearing."* Educators need to understand that trying to teach a child with autism to make eye contact may make processing auditory information more difficult. The child may not be able to process speech and gestures at the same time. But children with autism have other strengths that can be used for teaching, such as touch, visuals (pictures, words, videos), and music.

Teaching with Touch

We have many autistic adults who rely on someone to <u>talk</u> them through daily activities. Charles Hart wrote in **Without Reason** (1989) about his autistic brother and his autistic son. He said his mother would have to tell his brother what to do. She would *"provide direction for every single step of his day's activities from arising in the morning until going to bed at night."*

No one seems to appreciate the seriousness of this problem. In 2015, there was a newspaper report from Southern California, **"Special Needs Student found Dead on School Bus. May have been waiting for Instructions."** Paul was a nineteen years old autistic student and the family reported that the usual bus driver would say, *"Let's go Paul"*, and he would get off the bus. This day the usual driver was not present and did not give the verbal instructions, so Paul stayed on the bus. It was a hot day and by the time he was found, it was too late. Paul was dead.

For some children with autism, teaching through touch - without language – may be preferable, so they don't incorporate the speech with the skill or routine. The goal is for the child to function independently and reliance on verbal instruction prevents this independence. Temple Grandin in

147

The Way I See It (2008) states: *"If their visual and auditory systems are giving them jumbled information, they may rely more on touch."*

Drs. Itard and Seguin taught through the use of touch, often physically guiding children through the motions. As discussed in *Chapter 1*, **The Forgotten Past**, Dr. Itard reported that he was surprised at the benefit of training the sense of touch. He was able to help Victor distinguish hot and cold, roughness and smoothness. He had Victor practice comparing objects through the sense of touch, such as a stone and a chestnut.

Dr. Seguin in his book, **Idiocy and Its Treatment by the Physiological Method** (1866), described teaching a child to climb a ladder by physically guiding the child's hands and feet through the steps. This is done without verbalizing instructions to the child. This enables the child to get the feel of the movement.

Teaching without speaking is very difficult and challenging because we teach typical children by constantly talking to them. My educational consultant was a director of two group homes for children with autism and she said she sometimes had to put tape over a caretaker's mouth, because we normally teach children through language and it is very difficult to change this. But you are not teaching language and you do not want the child to incorporate the language into the routine.

Physical assistance is useful because it can be faded (stopped) quickly, so the child does not rely on it. Because children with autism can see and hear, we often assume they need to be taught through those senses, because we teach typical children that way. But Drs. Itard and Seguin (chapter one, *the Forgotten Past*) were the first to discover that sometimes we need to teach the child by physically guiding them through the motions. If the visual and auditory channels are weak – as with deficient mirror neurons – then the child does not learn effectively through observation and imitation, and we need to try to teach through a different channel.

When David had individual lessons to learn gymnastics, his coach would use this technique. For example, to learn how to do flips, she had him on a trampoline and physically flipped his body in the air. This helped him get the feel of the motion. This flip was transferred to his swimming lessons. When David went to the state Special Olympics event in swimming, he was the only participant to do a flip turn at the end of the lane. The audience reacted with surprise and appreciation.

Many young children with autism will benefit from being taught how to dress themselves and wash their hands with touch and this is explained in the next chapter. This accommodates the brain deficit of lack of observation and imitation and teaches to the strength of rote memory. The skill is broken into steps and taught the same way over and over.

Teaching with Visuals

The brain difficulties with memory and planning must be accommodated when communicating with children with autism. We often think if we have told the child where he is going (school, grocery store, zoo, therapy) then he "knows." Unfortunately, he may not be able to associate what you are saying with memory. He will then quickly forget what you said and not understand where he is going. To circumvent this deficit with short-term memory and associational memory, we focus on the child's strengths with visuals that give a picture that does not disappear.

I found it helpful to have small laminated pictures with a hole punched in the corner and kept on a clasp. David could hold it in his hand, so he had a reminder of where he was going. It is best if the picture is of the child at the destination site, because it creates more meaning from the child's perspective. Sometimes an object held in the hand can be useful, such as a toothbrush when going to the dentist, or a napkin or spoon when going to a restaurant or the shopping list (child's list) when going to the grocery store.

Moving is difficult for anyone, but can be extremely stressful for a child with memory difficulties and the inability to imagine the future. My husband was in the Air Force and we moved many times. We found the most effective way to assist David in understanding what was happening, was to provide him with pictures of his new environment prior to the move. One of us would have to go to the destination site to arrange housing, and take pictures of the house, McDonald's, Blockbuster Video, grocery store, swimming pool and his favorite restaurants. During the actual move, David sat in the back seat of the car with his pictures. In this way, we supported his mental perspective of always being in the present and he did not have to rely on memory or imagination.

When teaching skills, we often forget to support the lack of associative memory with a child with autism. David was thirteen years old and taking private lessons for gymnastics. The focus of instruction was on improving skills within each routine. When the coach tried to improve his form by telling him to *"Point your toes,"* David responded, *"I did,"* and he became more agitated with each correction.

In order for him to understand the criticism, he would have to imagine himself performing the skill by accessing associational memory. What if he could not bring up the memory or imagine himself performing the skill even though he had just done it? I brought a video camera to the next lesson and filmed David performing his skills. When the coach wanted to make a correction, I would rewind the tape. They could look at the monitor of the video camera and the coach could visually show David imperfections to be improved. This worked very well, because it circumvented the need for David to access associative memory.

Pictures can be used to communicate about something in the past or the future, but should be presented from the child's perspective. For example, pictures of the child doing various activities can support memory and help teach language meaningful to the child. The "memories" may be stored as visual pictures. I took pictures of David cutting the grass, taking out the garbage, cooking, and going for a run with his dad and this seemed to create more meaning for him by visually associating himself with various activities. As noted in the last section, the child may not remember that he knows how to do things he learned by rote.

In addition to supporting deficits in associational memory, visuals may enable the child to create his self-identity. A scrapbook can be created to include admission tickets, pictures or other souvenirs from various events into the book with the dates, thus creating a visual memory to support the lack of associational memory.

We must remember that we are not curing a deficit, but rather supporting a neurological impairment. Today, at age 32, David often has difficulty remembering what I ask him to do. For example, I asked him, *"David would you go into the storage room and get me the fan?"* I stood at the top of the stairs and the storage room was at the bottom of the stairs. He went into the storage room and then said, *"What am I looking for?"* I have a greater appreciation for the memory problem, as I often go into a room these days and can't remember why I am there!

Another area of brain strength in children with autism that may facilitate teaching may be reading and writing (or typing). Temple Grandin writes in **The Way I See It** (2008) *"In some nonverbal individuals, verbal language is impossible, but they learn to read and express themselves through typing. Their speech circuits are scrambled but they can still communicate through the typed word."*

There are patients who have pure word deafness that is caused by a lesion in the left hemisphere. This is the inability to comprehend spoken words. Yet, the patient can still read and understand writing (visually presented words). For example, a patient (W.B.) suffered a stroke and then he could read and write, but not speak. Despite a normal hearing test, he could not understand spoken language. The condition of "deaf but can hear" persisted for the rest of his life. Temple Grandin writes *"A child who has difficulty hearing auditory detail will benefit from the use of visual supports, such as written words on flash cards, written instructions, or written homework assignments."*

Even when teaching high functioning verbal children with autism, they may need visuals to assist with learning. Jennifer McIlwee Meyers wrote (2010) **How to Teach Life Skills to Kids with Autism and Asperger's** that *"When I was growing up, my parents expressed my chore list in the vaguest possible terms, and those only verbally."* Mrs. Meyers tells us she would have benefited from *"specific schedules, lists or chore charts."* This is an adult with Asperger's Syndrome telling us how we can help children on the autism spectrum. We often mistakenly assume that if children with autism have language, then they don't require written information.

Teaching with Music

Dr. Itard and Seguin in the first chapter noted that music was helpful with teaching children with autism. Temple Grandin writes in **Thinking in Pictures** (1995) *"Therapists have learned from experience that sometimes nonverbal children can be taught to sing before they can speak. In some people the brain circuits used for singing may be more normal than the circuits used for speech. Possibly the song rhythm helps to stabilize auditory processing and* *block out intruding sounds. This may explain why some autistic children use commercial jingles as an attempt to communicate."*

Unfortunately, we often forget the lessons from the past. In March 2016, the television news featured a family of a child with autism because they had "discovered" that music helped their child to speak. This is another area that researchers have generally ignored, perhaps because music is not used to teach typical children.

Music slows the words and helps emphasize the vowels and consonants, as well as the changes in pitch or tone. Some neuroscientists are beginning to study the use of music to teach children with autism. In 2010, Catherine Wan and Gorrfried Schlaug published an article on **Neural pathways for language in autism: the potential for music-based treatments**, promoting the theory that music training can facilitate language in otherwise nonverbal children with autism. They state *"Theoretically grounded music-based interventions have been underutilized, which is unfortunate because music perception and music making is known to be a relative strength of individuals with autism."*

Paul Arkoprovo and colleagues wrote an article in <u>Frontiers in Human Neuroscience</u> (2015) that their *"Findings suggest that sung directives may play a useful role in engaging children with ASD and also serve as an effective interventional medium to enhance socio-communicative responsiveness."* David was in preschool (1989-1992), and he had a teacher who would sing instructions to him. She was so effective that we decided to leave David (ages 4-7) in her classroom for several years, even though he was slightly older than the other children.

People who have had strokes and cannot speak often can sing and will understand speech better if you sing to them. Music is processed in a different area of the brain than speech. As noted previously, when one brain circuit is turned off, another one may turn on.

When David was young, I often had difficulties finding him in the house or the backyard, because he would not respond to my calling him. I started singing a song, *"Where is David, Where is David, Here I am, Here I am."* I discovered he would sing the song and I could then find him.

Teach "To Do" not "To Know"

Teaching children with autism in the regular classroom relies on verbal instruction and imitation. Yet, as Temple Grandin tells us in **The Way I See It** (2008) *"Young children with autism spectrum disorders do not learn by listening to and watching others, as do typical children. They need to be specifically taught things that others seem to learn by osmosis."*

In a classroom setting, we are usually teaching "to know", because we are teaching through symbolism and associative memory. For example, we may try to teach a child with autism to identify a color found in various objects. We expect the child to take the various details of objects of the same color and create an associative concept. This is teaching "to know" a concept.

But Temple Grandin tells us she associated meanings with actions. In **The Autistic Brain,** Dr. Grandin states: *"Unfortunately, today's educational system is letting these kids down. It's phasing out hands-on classes, like shop."* In **Thinking in Pictures**, she states it is important for children with autism to have structured activities both at home and at school, *"with lots of opportunity for interesting hands-on activities."* We need to teach hands-on experiences, such as arts and crafts, cooking, board games and recreation.

Typical children learn through language. They can read a story and imagine themselves in the role of different characters. Brain science informs us that typical children use mirror neurons to comprehend reading. They can imagine themselves doing what a character does in the story, because they can relate it to something in associative memory and build more memories. Children with autism only relate to something they can do, and do not imagine themselves doing something they only read about.

We need to understand the wide diversity of processing in the brain to understand why children with autism learn differently. We tend to think of brain deficits resulting in a complete loss of function, but usually it is a partial loss. Some children with autism can read (decode words), but fail to understand the meaning of what they read.

Decoding words is a rote memory function (strength in some children with autism) but combining meaning with sentences requires long distance connections and associative memory. The decoding of words occurs in one area of the brain and the meaning is processed in other areas. The child may know the meaning of some words in a sentence, but still not process the meaning of the sentence.

Neurology also explains how comprehension can be processed in different areas of the brain. Dr. Restak writes in **The Modular Brain: How new discoveries in neuroscience are answering age-old questions about memory, free will, consciousness and personal identity** (1994) *"spoken and written comprehension occurs in separate areas within the brain (and) this is of course not at all the way we think of comprehension."* Temple Grandin writes in **Thinking in Pictures** (1995) how she had to read out loud to improve her comprehension. It seems highly likely that Temple Grandin processed reading comprehension more through the auditory circuits of the brain. She writes in **The Way I See It** that a child with autism *"may need to hear and read the word at the same time for comprehension to take place."*

I cannot learn a foreign language by listening to it. I have to see the written words, before I can process the sounds. As Dr. Restak reported, spoken and written comprehension occurs in separate areas of the brain, so learning difficulties can reflect these differences in brain function.

Dr. Restak writes in **The Modular Brain** (1994) about a patient who *"lost the ability to extract meaning from a sentence despite a retained ability to understand the meaning of each of the words in isolation."* If a child with autism is only compared to normal development and we fail to understand the neurological impairment, we only teach to the deficit and fail to accommodate the deficit. When educators assume children with autism process information the same as typical children, then they fail to understand how they think and learn differently.

Dr. Restak in **The Modular Brain** (1994) describes a patient who could describe inanimate things, but failed to differentiate animals. He could not verbally define an animal, but when shown a picture, he provided an elaborate description. Dr. Restak reports: *"This discrepancy in performance between word definitions and picture descriptions argues against the idea of a single semantic system shared by all of the senses. Instead, it seems likely based on patients such as this, that the processing of information by the different senses involves different brain networks and meaning systems."*

Comprehending speech includes deciphering the words and having the brain connections to various areas of the brain to interpret meaning. We normally process verbal communication without hearing every word, because we are interpreting the gist or general meaning of the message. In addition, we often obtain clues to the message from the environment and physical gestures. For example, if the conversation is about cooking, then if one hears a word that sounds like "clothes" when it is actually "cloves," we can easily make the correction based on the meaning in the sentence.

The child with autism often attaches a meaning to a word, phrase or sentence, but the meaning is unique to the child. One day, David and I purchased lunch at a fast-food restaurant. As he was carrying his tray to the table, he dropped his tray and said *"Robber, robber."* Of course, this is not something the staff wanted to hear in a public place! They graciously replaced David's lunch (probably to shut him up). Temple Grandin reported she would fly a kite as a young child, and when it hit the ground, she would say *"persecution."*

One day, David came into the room where I was and he said *"Green screen."* Since I did not understand what he was saying, I put my hand in his and said, *"Come, show me."* We went to his playroom and I discovered he was having trouble playing his Wheel of Fortune game. When I got it working, I realized it had a green screen as a background.

We often think we have taught the child to greet someone, but soon discover the child focuses on a detail. The child may respond to *"How are you today?"* with *"I am fine today."* But the child may only respond if the complete request is made, including the word *"today."* If you don't include the word *"today,"* the child may not respond. This happens because their brains focus on details and fail to connect to the left hemisphere in the brain to interpret the general meaning of the sentence.

A child may focus on a detail such as the sound of the word rather than the meaning. David thought *"pieces of chicken"* was hysterical. He also likes homonyms, such as pair (pair of eyes), pare (pare an apple) and Maine, mane and main. If a sentence contains one of these words, he becomes focused on the word and not the meaning of the sentence.

Just like split-brain patients, children with autism can learn a meaning to a word, but have difficulties associating more than one meaning to that word. We can teach the words "up" and "down," but meanings of words can change easily such as "get down," "step down," "calm down," "back down," or "put down." The word "up" can be "clean up," "get up," "mess-up," "dress up," "pick up," or "fed up." When we understand the brain deficits, then we can help the child adapt to the world.

Children with autism often repeat dialogue from movies, books or television that they have listened to repeatedly and memorized. This speech seems quite sophisticated, but is actually a reflection of their strong rote memories and attempts to associate meaning with it.

One evening the electricity went off and David came running into the room and said, *"Does anyone know any scary ghost stories?"* This initially struck us as quite funny, but David was not trying to tell a joke. We have to look at the communication based on the context. He was repeating a sentence from a book we often read for him and this meant, *"Why did the lights go out?"*

The child with autism will often repeat something just said. If I ask a child, *"Do you want peaches or pears?"* he will respond *"peaches or pears."* This is called immediate echolalia. But labeling behavior does not explain it. Brain science teaches us that the child with autism has memory difficulties and cannot imagine a peach or pear. Therefore, we have to remember to put the items in front of him, so he can choose. It might be easier for the child to "point" to what he wants.

A behavior often observed in individuals with autism is called perseveration on a response that can be either verbal or behavioral. David often responds to what I say with, *"Good idea."* It sounds good until you have heard it a dozen times in one day. He also says, *"You have pretty blue eyes."* It can get so repetitive that we have to limit it to one time per day. Perseveration on a response is common in patients with frontal lobe damage in the brain. In children with autism, the lack of connections to the frontal lobe can result in the same type of behaviors.

Another language characteristic of children with autism is reversal of pronouns, substituting *"you"* for *"I."* The child may say, *"You want juice."* Using names will help create understanding for the child for it keeps identification specific (details). For example, say, *"David is cutting with scissors"* or *"David, throw the ball to Mommy."*

The child with autism has difficulty associating meaning with words and more difficulty when the words can refer to different people. An article by Science Daily, titled **"New Brain Imaging Research Reveals Why autistic Individuals Confuse Pronouns"** reports, *"errors in choosing a self-referring pronoun reflect a disordered neural representation of the self, a function processed by at least two brain areas – one frontal and one posterior."* The lack of long-distance connections in the brain may make it difficult for the child to process the different meanings of pronouns. The use of pronouns shift based on who is speaking.

When I started taking pictures of my son doing things, showing these pictures to him and narrating his accomplishments, he seemed to develop an autobiographical memory of himself as an individual with talents and the ability to do things by himself. When he became a boy scout at age 9, I showed him a picture of his Dad in a scout uniform, but it had no meaning for him. When I took pictures of David in his scout uniform, he would smile and seemed quite excited about it. We have to remember to teach from the child's perspective.

Teaching Meaningful Communication

Meaningful communication for a child with autism is taught by: 1) combining speech or gestures with actions; 2) using the child's interests; and, 3) teaching communication in a variety of environments that enable the child to get his needs met.

1. Combine words with actions.

The goal for teaching children with ASD is different than the goal for teaching typical children because they think and learn differently. We need to teach children with autism "to do," and that includes communication. They need to know when and how gestures and words will help them get their needs met. We do this by pairing the communication with their actions.

One does not teach skills and language at the same time. Once skills are learned, language can be modeled based on what the child is doing. I found having frequent family meals together was an opportunity to teach language in a meaningful way. By putting food in serving bowls, it creates the need to ask for what you want or ask someone to pass something to you. It is a time to describe what you are doing, such as *"I am eating with a fork"* and *"Please pass the salt to me."* This teaches meaning through activity. Once a child has learned an activity, such as setting the table, then we can teach language by describing what the child is doing, such as *"I am putting the fork on the left side of the plate and the knife and spoon on the right side of the plate."*

When David is reading recipes, he sometimes encounters words he does not understand. This is a great opportunity for him to learn words in a meaningful and contextual way. A recipe for corn muffins states, *"For maximum crown on muffins let the batter rest for 5 minutes."* He understood a crown was something worn on the head, so I explained that the crown on a muffin would be the head or top of the muffin. Children with autism have enough difficulties applying one meaning to a word, so we have to remember two different meanings can be a greater challenge.

Another time while cooking, David was confused by the term, *"crimp the crust."* This is a great way to teach language, since the meaning can be combined with the action and the child's interest.

2. Use Child's Interests

Communication has to be meaningful from the child's perspective, which is quite different from how most of us communicate. David would repeat television commercials, such as *"Bring out the Hellman's (mayonnaise), bring out the best."* To make the phrases communicative, he needed to learn to use them in a manner useful for getting his needs met. At the dinner table, if we ask David to, *"Please pass the mayonnaise,"* he will pass the mayonnaise while saying *"Bring out the Hellman's, bring out the best."* If we ask him to *"please pass the butter,"* he will respond with *"You butter believe it."* He also likes *"I'm using a dollop of Daisy (sour cream)."* Teaching strategies need to include basic words or phrases that are meaningful to the child and are useful for him to get his needs met in a variety of environments.

When David was a child, he would answer "yes" to any question asked. He understood a reply was expected, but he failed to understand the meaning of the question. The challenge is to find real-life situations where pairing the question with his response would create meaning for him. For example, when riding in the car, we would ask him if he needed to use the toilet, just as we were pulling off the highway. Of course, he said "yes" and we stopped so he could use the toilet. Repeating this scenario numerous times resulted in his understanding through rote memory.

When we teach typical children to read, we expect them to learn about the world through reading. When teaching children with autism, we have to be more specific with our teaching goals and consider where it will benefit the child to reach greater independence as an adult. The goal then becomes trying to make reading meaningful (functional) for the child by using the child's interests. Reading can help with instructions for a game, a recipe for cooking, following a schedule, reading aisle signs in a grocery store to locate products, or reading a menu.

When teaching reading comprehension to David, it had to be related to something he was doing, so it had meaning for him. He could not relate to what someone else was doing. He played computer games, so he read game strategies and this made sense to him. With cooking, he reads each step of the recipe as he cooks. Even if he has made the recipe many times, he still reads each line. This avoids the need for reliance on memory and enables him to keep the sequence of steps correct.

When teaching math, I used objects David could physically manipulate to count, add, multiply, etc. When he made hash browns, he lined up three rows of eight hash browns. This created an opportunity to teach multiplication in a real-life situation.

I created word math problems that would be meaningful to him: "*You rented a game at Blockbuster Video for $4.29. You gave the store clerk a five dollar bill, how much change did you receive?*" Academics have to be embedded into activities the child with autism does in the community and at home.

Some children have motor difficulties learning to write and their handwriting is slow and difficult, so using a computer may be helpful. For some children, printing and writing will be two different languages and writing may be easier, because the words are connected. Most children with autism are comfortable with a computer and this can be useful for Email, text messaging or word processing.

Practical applications for writing include making lists of things he wants for his birthday or Christmas or making shopping lists. Learning to sign one's name is beneficial, because there are many instances where this is necessary, such as obtaining identification cards, or setting up a bank account. Being able to write one's name sends a message that he is literate.

3. Teach in a variety of environments

Temple Grandin has been telling us for decades that children with autism need to get out into the world. She writes in **The Way I See It** (2008) *"I think many parents and educators coddle their children with ASD (Autism Spectrum Disorder) far more than they should. Children with ASD don't belong in a bubble, sheltered from the normal experiences of the world around them."* Teaching children to function in a classroom does not teach them to function in the community. We need to teach "to do" rather than "to know."

History and brain science have shown that children with autism do not learn through observation and imitation. This means that every time they go into a different environment, they are unable to attribute meaning to what they see, so they fail to learn from their environment. Therefore, we have to teach them how to function in a variety of environments by using their strengths.

Drs. Itard and Seguin reported that children with autism need to use objects in real-world environments. Teaching a child to label a grocery cart is not going to teach him to push it through the store or to understand the purpose of the store. Everything has meaning only from the child's perspective, so he has to actually perform skills where they are useful.

Typical children go into a grocery store and observe a parent pushing a grocery cart, putting groceries into the cart and paying for the groceries. Young children want to imitate adults, so there are often mini carts available, so the child can imitate Mom and push a cart herself. The child with autism may focus on a crack in the floor, so he is not learning about the environment through observation and imitation. The child needs to be directed to expected behaviors in every environment. In a grocery store, this starts with the child holding the handle on the grocery cart and putting a few groceries into the cart. Chapter 11 explains specifically how to teach in the community. We don't teach typical children in this manner, because they seem to learn by osmosis.

Social Skills

Most people value social situations with emotional connections to others. It is such an important part of our lives that it is difficult to understand someone who does not have this drive for social connections. Often parents and educators want children with autism to have greater social lives. Temple Grandin stated in her book, **Thinking in Pictures**, *"Sometimes parents and professionals worry too much about the social life of an adult with autism. I make social contacts via my work. If a person develops her talents, she will have contacts with people who share her interest."*

The social skills important for children with autism relate to proper manners and kindness to others. Jennifer McIlwee Myers discusses how to teach these social skills to children with autism in several chapters of her book (2010), **How to Teach Life Skills to Kids with Autism and Asperger's.** She describes how her father taught her to shake hands, teaching to the details of strength of grip, how long to hold the grip, and when and where a handshake is used. He also taught the skill repeatedly and in various environments, where it would be used. In other words, he taught to details and rote memory and generalized the skill to other environments.

Mrs. Myers discusses that what is taught is important, although the way a skill is taught may vary based on the child's needs, such as use of pictures, short phrases, or written instructions. She very adequately describes how to teach children with autism to be kind to others in various circumstances and I highly recommend her book.

Parents and teachers can learn from this type of information from those who think and learn differently and are able to tell us about it. Most teachers understand typical child development, but have no knowledge of what needs to be taught to children with autism. They often associate social skills with normal development and try to teach how to have a conversation, ask questions, engage a peer in play, and how to observe and imitate others. We can't change a neurological deficit, so the goal is to enable the person with autism to learn skills - such as board games, bowling, swimming, and arts and crafts – that give structure to enable him to be around others in a variety of environments.

The family is the first social environment and children with autism need to learn to be part of the family. Having autism does not excuse one from having proper manners or doing family chores contributing to the family. This provides the basis for becoming an adult with proper manners, who contributes to society. Even the youngest member of the family is often able to put napkins on the table. It is easier to teach the proper way to behave early, rather than to change behavior that may have become entrenched over the years.

Behaviors as Communication

It is inappropriate to interpret observed behavior in children with autism as lack of motivation, or not paying attention, or an attempt to avoid the learning situation. Teachers and caretakers interpret behaviors in children with autism compared to normal development and not based on the different thinking and learning in autism. Since our children appear "normal," we interpret their behavior based on our own brain perspective of the world. We often are too controlling and try to direct behaviors before understanding the behavior from the child's perspective. When we begin to understand how children with autism think and learn differently, then we can respond differently.

The onus of communication falls on the parent or caretaker. Individuals with autism understand language differently and use language differently. We have to adjust our communication to their perspective. We also have to interpret their behaviors as a form of communication, because they cannot tell us what the problem is and they may not know themselves.

The teacher needs to go slowly and not try to teach too much at one time. If the child has aberrant behaviors, consider the following possibilities: 1) Are you providing enough support for the child? Are there enough visuals to guide the child? 2) Are you trying to teach two things at the same time – such as skills and language? 3) Is the environment too crowded or distracting? 4) Is the child not feeling well?

Examples are always helpful. David was nine years old and enjoyed going to the ice cream store every week. After having his ice cream, he would choose what flavor he would have the next week. One day, he entered the store and they did not have the flavor he was expecting to order. He became upset, pacing the floor and mumbling to himself. I thought he might have a meltdown. The clerk took me aside and told me she had the flavor in the freezer. I thanked her, but told her, *"No, I want David to have a chance to handle this himself."*

I sat down and asked David, *"Would you like to sit down?"* He sat down. I waited a few moments and asked him, *"Do you want to choose another flavor?"* He answered, *"No."* I waited a few moments and asked, *"Would you like to leave now?"* He walked out the door.

Most children would not turn down an opportunity to have an ice cream, but for children with autism, the need for sameness and predictability is more important than an ice cream treat. David learned a valuable lesson that day, and he never again decided what he would have to eat, until he was able to *"see what they have available."*

Every environment will present unique challenges. We often try to placate our children so they don't have a meltdown in public, but if we allow an accommodation, the child will expect the same accommodation the next time. For example, like many children with autism, David would only eat on one size plate. When he started eating in a cafeteria, he did not have control over the size of the plate. The desserts and bread are put on a small plate. One day, David chose a dessert. It sat on the table and David would not touch it. I was thankful that he did not start screaming, because of the small plate. If he had, I would have removed the dessert, rather than try to accommodate him.

Although I could have gotten a large plate or a take-out box, he would expect a large plate every time he came to the cafeteria, so I try not to make special accommodations for him. When we left, the dessert was sitting on the table and nothing was said. There are not many children who will reject a dessert! The next time we went to the cafeteria, he knew what to expect and he accepted the dessert on a small plate. We have to be careful that we don't intervene too quickly to make things okay. The child with autism has a differently wired brain and it takes more time for them to adjust to and accept minor changes.

Children with autism sometimes get labeled as "runners," and the focus is on how to stop the behavior. But brain science teaches us that we need to look at the behavior from the child's perspective. Some children may not be running away, but running toward something of interest. In the drug store, David would run to the hair color area, where he could touch the hair swatches. The goal is to retain the child's interest in the hair samples, but shape the behavior into something more appropriate than running through the store. When I was training David to shop in various community environments, I included *"touch hair"* to the bottom of the shopping list. The first time training in the store, we only shopped for one item and headed to the hair samples for his reward. Once he understood that he would get to his item of interest, he became more patient.

We often make the mistake of thinking that when the child gets older, he will be able to learn like typical children. David was a teenager and taking private gymnastics lessons and after a few lessons, he started dropping to the ground and not following instructions. Rather than viewing it as noncompliant behavior, we need to view it from the condition of autism. How is he to understand the meaning of the activity, when he has a mirror neuron deficit? Are we trying to teach through too many sensory channels? The coach and I established a written list of skills to be done and how many of each. David could check off each skill when he completed it. This reduced the need for extensive verbal instructions and provided a sense of meaning and structure to the activity. Whenever the child reacts with aberrant behaviors, we need to consider what we may have done wrong and try again.

Dr. Edouard Seguin wrote in the 1800's that if we should cause stress to the child, we should remember it is our fault and take the child for music or exercise. I find his advice spot on. We often expect children with disabilities to perform many hours per day and to behave better than typical children. When typical children cry or resist, we often attribute it to their being tired or not feeling well, but when children with disabilities resist, we place the blame on the child as willfulness.

The ability of children to learn by rote has been recognized for years. Temple Grandin wrote in **Thinking in Pictures** (1995) *"Autistic children need to learn everything by rote."* The National Research Council (2001) wrote in **Educating Children with Autism** *"The ability to learn material by rote may be less impaired than that involved in the manipulation of more symbolic materials."* So one has to wonder why we continue to try to teach children with autism through symbolism (language) or "show and tell."

So how do we teach children "to do" by rote? Rote learning consists of breaking a task into steps (details) and repeating the steps until you no longer have to think about it, because it becomes automatic. We learn many things through rote memory, such as multiplication tables, tying shoes, playing the piano or riding a bike. We can also teach children with autism routines of behavior in a variety of environments, including chores, shopping, eating in restaurants, recreation skills and job skills through rote learning. Rote learning is structured and it is teaching "to do" rather than "to know."

The next three chapters will show you how to teach a child with autism through rote memory and in a variety of environments. I will also discuss how to create structure in the home to help the child understand what behaviors are required in each area.

Chapter 10

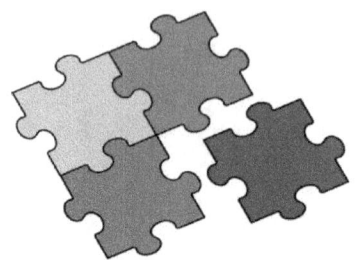

Teaching Self-Care and Chores

"Tell me and I forget. Teach me and I remember. Involve me and I learn." Benjamin Franklin.

Self-care skills should be a priority for teaching young children with autism, because it helps the child understand that he is capable of doing something and it reduces the reliance on adult direction (if it is done correctly). Self-care skills are part of learning independence and other children learn these skills much earlier than a child with autism, because they observe and imitate, but our children must be specifically taught. Self-esteem, independence and self-reliance are built on the ability of the child to provide his own care, including doing laundry, fixing meals and numerous other chores.

Teaching skills to children with autism is most effective if it is visual (supports memory deficits), meaningful (to the child) and contextual (in the environment where the skill is used). Children with autism have strengths with rote memory and attention to detail. Therefore, we teach skills by breaking the details into steps and repeating the steps over and over until it is established in rote memory.

C.H.O.R.E.S. Strategy

I consider all activities for children with autism as "chores." To discuss how to teach each task, I will use the mnemonic C.H.O.R.E.S. as a guideline. This may help you understand what you are teaching and why you are teaching it from the child's perspective. First, I will give you a general view and then use the same technique to show you how to teach each task.

C. Charts. Chores are broken into steps because the child attends to the details and learns by rote. There needs to be a clear beginning and ending. For example, washing hands begins with turning on the water and ends with turning off the water. What about drying the hands? That is a separate skill because it could be a towel, paper towel (pull or motion-detector), or automatic dryer (push button or motion-detector) and these are all details that must be specifically taught. Grocery shopping begins with getting the cart and ends with putting the cart away in the corral.

H. Have success in plan. Simplify the task so it does not overwhelm the child. You can't teach everything at once. For example, when we started teaching David to make the bed, we used a simple cover over a quilt that served as a sheet. He simply needed to pull the quilt over the pillows. When he was older, we taught him to put sheets on the bed and remove the sheets to wash. In addition, you want to use the child's interests whenever possible. For example, when you start teaching in a grocery store or restaurant, use his food choices. You don't want to change too many things at one time.

O. _Organize Materials and Simplify Instruction._ The child with autism has difficulties with associational memory so we need to collect materials needed for a task because this accommodates the deficit and reduces the need for language instruction. Materials for cleaning the house, washing a car, or cooking can be organized in a pail or specific area for the child. Instruction needs to be simplified, such as a simple left to right (L-R), top to bottom (T-B) for window washing, car washing, vacuuming or sweeping the floor. The child may need written instructions, rather than being told what to do, so he doesn't have to rely on memory. Many children with autism like numbers so a task can be structured with counting.

R. _Rely on child's learning strength to teach the activity._ Are you teaching through the child's sensory strength – vision, touch, or music? For example, when we taught David to cut the grass, we put his hand (touch) on the tall grass and then on the cut grass to indicate what the machine does that he is pushing around the yard. In addition, we created the boundaries (visual) of where to cut the grass. Initially, I cut one row around the outside of the area to be cut. Later, we had edging material around the flowerbeds so he cut to the edging material. If the child is not cooperating with your teaching, you may need to try a different approach to help the child understand what behaviors are expected.

E. *Every skill needs to generalize*. Once the routines is learned then it needs to be taught in a variety of environments, because details in each environment will be different and the child does not generalize easily to another environment. After teaching David self-care skills, we were staying at a motel. I discovered he used the soap with the plastic covering and used a bath mat to dry himself. He had to be taught to function in a variety of environments.

When teaching a skill, consider where that skill can be used to increase independence in other environments. For example, if the child is taking his food to the table on a tray at home, he can also do that at a fast-food restaurant or cafeteria.

S. *Strive for independence*. Too many adults with autism require someone to talk them through daily routines, because they have incorporated language as part of the skill. This is not independence. In order to avoid this problem, you should teach without language through touch or with visuals and limited language.

With instructional charts, parents and educators can quickly evaluate whether the child can perform the skill independently and where they need further instruction. Evaluation of progress is easy. You can stand back and watch the child independently perform the skill. If there are problem areas, then they are easily identified.

Because of the difficulties with generalization, the child should be taken to a different environment to determine if the skills transfer. If the child views the environment as different, he will not be able to perform the skill. We are not evaluating isolated school skills, but independent functioning in a variety of environments.

C.H.O.R.E.S. Hand washing

Let's start with a basic behavior of hand washing that is taught to young children. Here is the C.H.O.R.E.S. method:

C. **_Chart._** Hand washing is broken down into steps that need to be taught the same way each time. Anyone who works with your child needs to know the hand washing steps. They are to be performed in the same sequence, because you are teaching to rote memory. If the child needs any physical assistance, you can indicate this, but be sure to fade any assistance as soon as possible. Emphasize to teachers and caretakers that there should be NO TALKING during this routine.

HAND WASHING STEPS

1. Turn on water	_6. Rub right hand over left hand for count of four_
2. Wet Hands	_7. Rinse hands_
3. Push lever to get soap	_8. Turn off water_
4. Rub hands together for count of four	_9. Dry with towel (paper towel dispenser or automatic dryer)_
5. Rub left hand over right hand for count of four	

H. **_Have success in place._** Place your hands over the child's hands. You are going to put his hands through the motions of each step. Having a chart that provides the steps to be followed by anyone teaching the skill will help create success.

O. **_Organize materials and simplify instruction._** If there is the possibility of the water being too hot, you may be able to place a mark to indicate how far to turn the water on. When he is rubbing his hands together, you can structure each step by counting to four, because this helps the child understand how long the step lasts. After a few times, you want to stop counting, but continue the step with four motions, because you don't want the child to rely on someone to do it for him.

Each child is different, but within a few lessons, you should feel his hands respond to the motions and this is when you keep your hands close by his hands, but allow him to do the motion. As soon as possible, move your hands back by his elbows. This enables you to give him a gentle push on the elbow, if he stops doing the steps. Some people use pictures/words of the steps, but I would try to avoid this, as it may result in reliance on a support. Our goal is always independence. The visual or list of steps will be helpful if someone else is also teaching your child this skill, and you want them to do it in the same manner.

R. *Rely on child's learning strengths to teach activity.* Hand washing is taught through touch and rote memory learning.

E. *Every skill needs to generalize.* Every environment will have different soap dispensers, towel dispensers or electric hand dryers. Some will have water that turns on automatically, when your hands are put under the faucet. All these details have to be taught to the child, because they do not learn by observation and imitation. They are learning by doing, so they must experience hand washing in many different environments to accomplish generalization.

S. *Strive for independence.* I suggest a pump soap dispenser, because that is what one usually encounters in most public restrooms and you will be transferring the skill to other places. Remember that there is **no talking** while teaching the task, because you don't want the child to rely on someone to talk them through the task.

C.H.O.R.E.S. Dressing

I will share with you my experience teaching David to dress himself using the C.H.O.R.E.S. method.

C. *Chart.* First, we break the skill or task into steps. I posted the steps on the bathroom mirror, so I could follow the sequence. Because you are teaching to rote memory, it is important to follow the steps in the same sequence and teach it over and over until the child does not have to think about it. The steps are for the teacher's use, and not the child's. I found dressing skills the most difficult skill to teach (perhaps because David and I were both new at it) and teaching other skills became faster and easier.

H. *Have Success in the Plan.* Whenever possible, you want to simplify a skill, so the child can do it independently. For example, when initially teaching David to dress himself, I used pants with elastic waistbands, pullover shirts, tube socks and shoes with Velcro fastening. As long as you remember that the goal is independence, you can find strategies to enable the child to do it for himself.

O. *Organize Materials and Simplify Instruction*. At first, the child is not going to choose or organize his clothes to wear, so you want everything you need ready. You also want to decide where the teaching is going to take place. I chose the bathroom, because it gave me more control over my son's behaviors and prevented him from running away. Instruction is going to be hand-over-hand without speaking.

R. *Rely on Child's Learning Strengths*. The steps are taught by standing or sitting behind the child and placing your hands over the child's hands to guide them through the motions. This is hard work and takes some time. I put David's thumbs on the inside of the waistband for underwear and pants. He started by sitting in front of me and I guided him to put on the underwear and pants to his knees. Then, he stood up and finished pulling them up to his waist. I put the pull-on shirt on the counter in the proper position then guided one arm at a time into the sleeves. Finally, I put his hands on the bottom edge of the shirt and pulled his arms over his head. I had David sit down again to put on the socks and shoes, with me guiding his hands.

Gradually, the child will begin to use his hands and you should begin to decrease your assistance. Once he starts dressing himself, keep your hands at elbow level. In this way, if he does not initiate the next step, you are ready to push his arms toward the next item of clothing.

When teaching David to dress, I started out keeping my mouth closed, but eventually slipped back into verbal instructions. Soon, I discovered he would stand like a statue, waiting for me to verbally direct him. I told him to put on his shirt and he did it, and then stood patiently waiting for the next instruction. I returned to physical assistance and pushed his arm toward the next article of clothing. I learned my lesson: physical prompts can be faded, but verbal instruction cannot. After dressing, we both headed to the kitchen for breakfast, as this was our reward for hard work.

How quickly the child learns skills will depend on several factors such as: 1) The skill of the teacher which improves with experience; 2) Consistency in providing instruction time until the skill is embedded into rote memory; and 3) The level of mental retardation which indicates how fast the brain processes information. We all tend to want a quick fix and become impatient with a child who learns slowly, but if you do it for the child, then he will never reach the degree of independence you are seeking.

172

E. *Every Environment is Different.* Once the child has learned the task, it has to be generalized to other environments because details will differ in other environments and the child attends to the details. When David was eight-years old, he started going to a swim club where he changed clothes at the club. Fortunately, there was a room where I could accompany him. He had no problems taking off his clothes and getting his bathing suit on, but after swimming, the clothes were inside out and he could not straighten them. I realized that at home, he took his clothes off and put them in the laundry basket, so it had not been an issue. I then had to teach him to turn the clothes right side out. We often forget that everything has to be taught and everything has to be specific.

S. *Strive for Independence.* In our fast paced life, we often become impatient for the child to do the routine and it seems easier to do it for him. It is certainly quicker at the time to do things for the child, but we are not helping the child toward independence if we do not expect and demand (and wait!) for the child to do it himself. Don't do something for the child that he is capable of doing for himself. Children with autism do not take the initiative to do for themselves and will easily allow someone to do things for them. A normally developing child will state, *"I can do it myself,"* but the child with autism may not remember that he knows how.

Once the child learns the basic routine, he will have to learn how to lay out his clothes (back versus front), use buttons, zippers, and belts, and tie shoes. The dressing routine is slow and parents have limited time and energy. Therefore, I found it easier to incorporate teaching of skills at different times. For example, teaching buttoning or zipping can be incorporated when the child is putting on a jacket to go outside. Once the skill is learned, then it can be added to the morning dressing routine.

Behaviors with Self-Care

When we have taught self-care skills, we often think our job is finished, but there will be situations where some judgment is required. For example, during the process of David learning to dress himself, he learned a rule that the tags go in the back. One day, I found him wearing a bathing suit on backwards. Closer inspection revealed the only tag was on a pocket that was on the front of the bathing suit, so he followed the rule and put the tag in the back. I was able to explain to him that the rule did not apply to this bathing suit.

On occasion, I have discovered my son wearing clothes too large or too small for him. One day, he was wearing a pair of my husband's pants. Although they were several sizes too big for him, he held them up with a belt. He looked like Tom Hanks in the movie, **Big,** when he was transforming from an adult to a child. We can only hope that we encounter enough situations to create adult independence.

One morning, we were going for our morning walk and David showed up in his long underwear. I had told him the mornings were getting warmer and we would not need as many layers of clothing, so he decided he did not need his sweat pants and sweat shirt. It is a reminder that we tend to give general explanations rather than specifics!

I explained to him that this was "underwear" and is to be worn under other clothes for added warmth. I told him to take the long underwear off and put the sweat clothes on. I find it best to try to maintain a sense of humor during these unexpected situations.

I learned to be more specific in my instructions. For example, I showed him the outside thermometer and gave him guidelines such as 1) If temperature is 45 degrees or less, wear long underwear and sweatpants and sweatshirt; 2) If the temperature is between 45 and 65, just wear sweatpants and sweatshirt; 3) If the temperature is 65 or higher, you can wear shorts. This gave him a concrete visual way of deciding what to wear without me telling him. If we keep our sights on adult independence, then we can find ways to help the child make his own decisions.

Schedules for Self-Care

In addition to dressing skills, you must teach the child to brush his teeth, wash his face, wash and comb his hair and take a shower or bath. Every skill is broken down into steps and the skills are put together to create a complete routine for self-care. Once the child learns the routine, he does not have to be told what to do and he does not have to remember, because it is established in rote memory.

Schedules enable the child to know what to expect, and help him do the routine independently, without being told what to do. Although a parent may be doing most of the care for the child, you want to establish the schedule, before the child can do it all independently. This is where a visual schedule (picture/words) can be useful to help the child learn the routine. The child will become more cooperative, when he can understand what is going to happen and when.

Example of a Morning Schedule

1. Go to toilet	*8. Brush teeth*
2. Wash hands	*9, Wash face*
3. Make bed	*10. Comb hair*
4. Remove Pajamas; Fold Pajamas and place beside bed pillow	*11. Toilet*
5. Get dressed	*12. Wash hands*
6. Breakfast	*13. Check calendar for daily events*
7. Put dishes in sink	

Example of an Evening Schedule

1. Remove clothes	*10. Step out of shower*
2. Put clothes into hamper	*11. Take towel and dry off; top to bottom; front and back*
3. Use toilet	*12. Hang towel on rack*
4. Turn on shower to visual marker	*13. Put on pajamas*
5. Get into shower	*14. Brush teeth*
6. Rub soap on washcloth	*15. Comb hair*
7. Wash top to bottom; front and back	*16. Give Mom and Dad hug and kiss goodnight*
8. Run water over body, top to bottom; front and back	*17. Turn on music*
9. Turn off water	*18. Get into bed*

C.H.O.R.E.S. Method for Self-Care Schedules

C. *Charts.* I have included examples of morning and evening schedules.

H. *Have success in plan.* Since the goal is independence, there may be parts of a skill or task that require additional structure/information, so you don't have to tell the child when to start and stop an activity. For example, how long should one brush his teeth or take a shower? Some electric or battery operated toothbrushes will have a two-minute timer built into them, that buzzes when the two minutes is over. For a shower, the child may not know when it is over. You can use a kitchen timer or a favorite song can be played. When the song is over, the shower is over. Another approach is to teach a washing routine that has a clear beginning and ending.

If the child is taking a bath, you need to find a way to indicate how much water to put in the tub. I used a colored marker on the bottom of the lever that closes the drain of the tub. In this way, the water level went to the bottom of the lever and then I faded the colored marker so the visual cue (lever) was part of the tub. A visual cue enables the child to focus on something specific to indicate the water level. In other words, the concepts have to be specific, literal, and concrete.

O. *Organize materials and simplify instruction.* Children with autism have difficulty with organization, so it is important to remember to have soap, shampoo, towels, etc. in a specified visible area for the child to complete the routine. They have been known to complete the routine without the use of these items, if they are not available. You can assume the child will not come ask you for something. At a later date, you can teach where extra supplies are stored and how to retrieve them as needed.

Does the instruction meet the child's needs so he does not rely on someone to tell him what to do and does he understand the process? If the child shows aberrant behaviors, consider what structures or support would help the child understand.

R. *Relate meaning to the activity.* Creating a routine of self-care skills done about the same time each day enables the child to know what behaviors are expected and when – thus creating meaning to the activity. The morning routine can be followed with breakfast as a reward for completing the task.

E. *Every Environment is Different.* The child with autism has to learn to generalize behaviors to different times and places. Whenever self-care skills will be needed in another environment, it is an opportunity to generalize the routine. You need to organize his supplies in a new environment to replicate the routine he was familiar with, such as hanging the towel on a bar and unwrapping a new bar of soap.

S. *Strive for Independence.* After a skill is learned, we have to teach when and where it is used, to facilitate independence. Once the skills are established in rote memory, it becomes easier to introduce some changes into the routine, such as taking a shower at a different time, or changing clothes for a specific occasion. This may require some advanced notice by telling him there will be a change and/or showing the change on his daily schedule.

C.H.O.R.E.S. Preparing Meals

C. *Chart* details of what you want to teach. Preparing meals can include setting the table and clearing the table, but you can't teach everything at once.

H. *Have Success in Plan.* Many children with autism have limited food choices when they are young and this is not the time to change the child's eating habits. For example, David ate tater tots for breakfast. He carefully lined the baking sheet with four lines of eight each. Don't get impatient and try to control every step. Independence is the goal so let him do some things his own way. Start with what they know. Also remember that the child cannot multitask so meal preparation will always be limited to one dish. Sometimes, when I prepare an evening meal, he will prepare the corn muffins from a box mix. If he prepares one item, I manage the rest.

O. **Organize Materials and simplify Instructions.** When the child is preparing a dish, make sure the tools and food items are available and in sight for the child, so he does not have to rely on associative memory. Try to teach one thing at a time. For example, you can prepare the waffle batter, and the child can use the correct ladle size to pour batter into the waffle maker.

R. **Relate Meaning.** To make a task meaningful, we need to use visuals, the child's interests and teach in the environment where it is needed. One day, I discovered David was making Pop Tarts and he would force the lever on the toaster to make them pop up. When I showed him how he could adjust the temperature on the toaster, he said *"They didn't say that on the box."*

Most recipes leave an important step out of the directions, such as when to turn the heat on the stove down. This requires some judgment, as an electric stove will be slower to cool down than a gas stove. A child with autism will follow the directions specifically and fail to make adjustments for the cooking temperature. I found it helpful to adjust the directions, so David would turn down the heat before the food burned.

It is always helpful to relate to the child's interests. David liked cheeseburgers without the bun, so I started teaching him to make his cheeseburger from a box of Hamburger Helper. When we went to the grocery store to buy a box of Hamburger Helper, David discovered there were other varieties and he decided he had to try all of them. This helped expand his meal choices. In addition, I showed him the Chicken Helper. This is a great way to slowly add change (new details) to a routine.

E. Every Environment is Different. Children with autism do not generalize routines to other environments so they have to be taught in a variety of environments. When we stay in a hotel that provides a breakfast buffet, this was an opportunity to have David prepare his own breakfast in a different environment. In addition to cereal, they often have a waffle maker and David enjoys waffles.

S. Strive for Independence. There are many simple ways to prepare food that enable a child to do it himself. Cookie dough simply needs to be cut or scooped and put on a cookie sheet to be baked in the oven. There are numerous microwave items with easy to follow instructions. Instruction books need to be very specific and visual for the child to follow. We must always remember the goal is for the child to do it himself and not depend upon someone telling him what to do.

Daily and Weekly Schedules

The child needs visual daily and weekly schedules, so he begins to learn what is expected. Some tasks are not performed daily, but need to be incorporated into routines so the child knows when to include the activity or task, such as cutting nails and washing hair. These activities can be scheduled on weekly chore day since they are done only once a week.

Mark a calendar with pictures/words indicating the main activity for the day, such as swimming, school, or community shopping. David and I would review the calendar every day, and he would mark the day with an "X". The child also needs a constant visual - to act as memory - until he gets to his destination. It can be an object or a picture such as the swim bag with bathing suit and towel to take to swimming, or a grocery list for shopping. We often assume if we have told the child where he is going, he will remember, but this is often not the case. Children with autism may not be able to access associative memory, so routines enable the child to understand what is going to happen and when.

Non-structured Environments

Parents and teachers need to be cautioned that children with autism do not function well in unstructured environments, because they do not observe and imitate and do not connect social meaning to what they see. Because children with autism perceive the world differently, it is difficult for caregivers to understand how structure provides information that most of us interpret easily from looking at the environment.

Creating structure in the home makes it easier for the child to understand the purpose of each area, because each area is designed for a particular activity and one activity follows another. The areas should help define what activity is expected. For example, you want a separate table for eating from one used for arts and crafts. In this manner, the child begins to understand that when he sits at this table, it is for eating. Eating does not take place in another area of the house, such as an area for watching TV or using the computer or playing video games.

Unfortunately, I know of too many unstructured situations where a child with autism wandered away – often with disastrous results. When my son was in preschool with an aide, the aide failed to watch him when he was on the playground and he crawled over the fence into the street. Fortunately, he was rescued before getting hit by a car.

When David was four, I wanted to take him to the neighborhood park. I had a neighbor and friend who was also a parent of a child with classic autism. I took one of David's hands and Sandy took the other and we started toward the park. David started screaming loudly. Sandy told me to keep my head high and keep on walking. I was sure someone would call the police, perhaps thinking we were kidnapping this child, but the problem was he could not understand where we were going and I didn't know how to convey the meaning.

We made it to the park and David saw numbers for the exercise circuit. At each stop, he carefully inspected the number. Since he loves numbers, he became very willing to go the park to *see the numbers.* Unfortunately, he loved going so much that he would leave the house unattended. We put latches on the top of the doors, and he soon learned that this meant he could not leave the house. We also scheduled going to the park as part of his routine, so he understood he would get to do something he wanted to do.

Parents all want their children to be like other children and to play together, but as much as we might like our children with autism to join the other children in free play, it isn't about the parental needs, but the child's needs. They will often wander off, grab something from a table or demonstrate aberrant behaviors due to lack of structure. They need to know where to sit, where to stand and what behaviors are expected in every environment.

When we had neighborhood cookouts, I would direct David to sit at a table with a hand-held game or something else to occupy him. I would have loved for him to run and play with the other children, but with deficient mirror neurons, he did not understand what they were doing, and he could not connect meaning to their behavior. He was happy sitting at the table with his game, so play with other children reflected my wishful thinking.

If a child is going to an unstructured environment such as a zoo, he will need assistance to understand where he is going and what he is going to do. Often there is a map showing the trail and the location of animals, and many children with autism are excellent with maps and mazes. In addition, you can put pictures of animals on a clipboard or communication device, so the child can check off a box when he identifies the animal and perhaps he can count the number he sees or identify something about the animal (based on the abilities of the child). You should also indicate time for toilet and time for eating on the schedule.

Medical Visits

Medical clinics and dental offices are also unstructured environments that have no meaning to young children with autism. Children need specific training for handling medical visits. The TEACCH Carolina Living and Learning Center is a residential facility and training program for 15 adults with autism. Keri Waldrop, Residential Supervisor, published a short article called *"Using Visual Structure for Medical Appointments"*. She clearly describes the use of visual schedules -- with examples -- that will help a person with autism understand what is going to happen in order to reduce anxiety.

When I was trying to teach David to go to the dentist, I did it the hard way, because I did not know any better. I will share it with you so you may better understand why visual schedules can be helpful. I found a dentist who worked well with disabled children. Usually talking with other parents of children with autism will help you find a dentist. I found one who scheduled a series of appointments for my four-year-old son every couple weeks, at no charge.

On the first appointment, we made it from the waiting room to the hallway, where David dropped to the floor. Rather than carry him to the chair, the exam consisted of a quick look in the mouth, while he was on the floor. For the second appointment, David made it into the exam chair, for another brief look at the mouth.

After several more appointments, David knew more what to expect and easily walked to "his" exam chair and sat down. If you don't have an understanding of what will happen in an environment and you don't observe and imitate others, it can be very frightening to have a bright light shining in your face and someone sticking things in your mouth.

It is important to consider the sensory input in the environment and how to help the child accommodate to it. A pair of sunglasses in the dental chair will help block out the bright light, and the discomfort of having someone's face close to you. The child also needs time to examine the equipment that will vibrate, spray water and remove water from his mouth. It can be helpful to take a picture of the child in the dental chair. He can hold it in his hand the next time he is headed to the dentist, so he knows what to expect.

If I had known the importance of visual information to help David function in a medical environment, it would have been much easier. If you don't prepare the child to function in these environments, providing care may include putting the child to sleep and this is an unnecessary risk.

Summary of Teaching Strategies based on Brain Function

1. Teach through strong sensory channels and teach without language if the child incorporates the language into the routines. Some sensory channels in children with autism are weak, so we need to teach through the channel that enables them to learn. For many, learning is easier if taught through touch by guiding the child through the motions, or the use of music to sing instructions. Higher functioning children with language may still require visual supports to enable them to remember what to do and the sequence of steps.

2. Use C.H.O.R.E.S. strategy because it teaches to details and rote memory.

3. Provide structure with counting or simple instruction of "Left to Right" and "Top to Bottom."

4. Once children with autism are taught a routine, then they will be willing to add new small details (changes) to the routine. It is when we overwhelm their ability to understand each environment, and the behaviors expected in each environment, that we see aberrant behaviors. Dr. Seguin wrote two hundred years ago that if we cause stress to the child, we should remember that we are at fault, and provide more support and structure to help the child understand.

The next chapter will discuss how to teach life skills in community environments.

Chapter 11

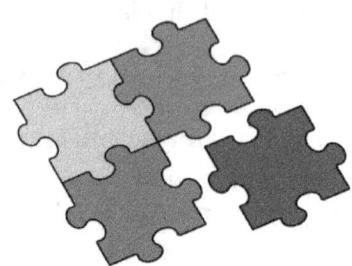

Teaching Life Skills in Community Environments

There is value in allowing others to learn, even if the task is not accomplished as quickly, efficiently, or effectively. Cheryl Merritt.

This chapter will discuss teaching chores, such as laundry and bed making, as well as functioning in a variety of community environments, such as grocery stores, cafeterias, sit-down restaurants and fast-food restaurants.

Every child with autism needs to learn the routines of daily living, including laundry and doing dishes. These are activities that the child needs to become more independent and self-sufficient as an adult. Public schools expect children with autism to learn like typical children, so they do not teach these skills. I know children with autism who can read and write, but can't take care of their personal needs, shop in a store, or fix a meal. Doing chores are job skills for kids. It teaches independence and responsibility.

A young child with autism can start by doing something simple such as taking his plate of food to the table. When he is finished eating, he carries the plate to the kitchen and places it on the shelf next to the sink. This behavior is meaningful and contextual. You will probably have to physically guide him through the activity rather than expect him to process language.

If the family is having a meal together, the child can start setting his place at the table with the plate, silverware, a napkin and drinking glass. You can use a placement with pictures of these items on it, so it becomes a matching task. To support the child's memory difficulties, put the items on the kitchen shelf where the child can pick them up and take them to the table, placing them in the proper position on the placemat. Initially, you may have to physically guide the child to indicate what you want him to do. Do not interject language until the skill is established in rote memory. Once the routine is established, you should remove the placement with the picture, so he does not rely on it.

After he can set the table for himself, he can learn to set the table for the entire family. He will need clear visual cues, such as the correct number of placemats and chairs at the table. Initially, you may have to physically guide him through it, counting the place settings as you go around the table touching each placemat. He can count the number of place setting and then count the number of plates, and number of utensils to set the table.

If he has a skill in one environment, you want to teach him when and where he can use that skill. At a fast food restaurant, he can take his tray of food to the table and when he is finished, he should take his tray to the trash can, empty his trash and then put the tray on top. By teaching the child what behaviors are expected in the environment, you avoid the situation of trying to teach what **not** to do.

If you are visiting grandparents, this is an opportunity to continue the skills, such as setting the table and taking his plate to the kitchen when he is finished. Try to recreate the routine as close to the original as possible and recognize the child may be distracted by the differences.

First, I will discuss teaching the child how to vacuum, do laundry, and make a bed and then show you how to incorporate chores into a schedule.

C.H.O.R.E.S. Vacuum

C. *Chart the steps of the chore.* First, tell the child he is going to "*Vacuum the floor*". Get the vacuum from the storage area (you will begin and end the skill with the vacuum in the storage area.

H. *Have Success in Plan.* The first time, take the child's hand to plug the machine into the wall, turn it on, pull it across the floor (no pattern), turn it off and unplug it. Return the vacuum to the storage area and praise the child for completing the chore. Let him put a sticker on his chart, something that is meaningful and interesting to the child – such as numbers, letters, or animals.

It may be difficult for the child to handle a cord and vacuum at the same time. Initially, I held the cord for David, while he concentrated on pushing the vacuum. Once he was able to maneuver the vacuum, I showed him how to hold the cord, so he would not run over it.

O. *Organize Materials and Simplify Instruction.* Many skills can be structured with the basic idea of left-to-right and top-to-bottom. You can give this instruction verbally and reinforce it as he actually does the skill. This helps the child focus. Otherwise, they tend to focus on a detail, such as making the footprints in the carpet disappear.

R. *Rely on Child's Learning Strengths*. A useful visual accommodation is to sprinkle white powder on the carpet and he is "vacuuming" it up. Showing the child how to empty the vacuum may help him understand what he is doing. Some children may benefit from a chart or picture of the steps to keep the sequence in order.

E. *Every Environment is Different.* Once the child can vacuum, he needs to know when and where this behavior occurs. The child needs the opportunity to do the task in a variety of environments because the machine will be different, the carpet or floor will be different and the room will be different. We are teaching to the details. When David had a volunteer job at a hospital cafeteria, he had to be taught to watch for people walking over the cord before moving the cord. He also had to be taught that when the machine did not work, he had to report to his boss.

S. *Strive for Independence.* Always remember the goal is for the child to perform the task by himself, so make sure he is not relying on verbal instruction or other cues from you.

C.H.O.R.E.S. Laundry

C. *Chart the Steps.* Chore starts and ends with basket.
1. Separate clothes for hot/cold into marked basket.
2. Move clothes from one basket into the machine. Close door.
3. Put soap and softener into dispenser.
4. Start machine. Set Timer.
5. When timer buzzes, transfer washed clothes to dryer.

6. Start dryer. Set Timer.

7. When timer buzzes, check clothes for dryness. If not dry, restart dryer and reset timer.

8. If clothes are dry, clean out filter and remove clothes to basket.

H. Have Success in Plan. Doing laundry requires many steps that cannot be taught all at once. We want to help the child understand the basic routine without becoming overwhelmed. Initially, I separated the clothes into baskets that were the correct size for one load. David moved the clothes from the basket into the washer (I had already added the detergent) and he turned on the washer. I used a kitchen timer, so he would know when to return to his chore. The child may enjoy putting a sticker on his chore chart when he completes the chore.

O. *Organize Materials and Simplify Instruction.* You want to provide easy access to soap, softener, baskets, measuring device and timer. Every step requires plans to teach in a manner that does not require the child to make a judgment. How are you going to teach how much laundry to put into the machine? The solution needs to be concrete and preferably visual. Most detergents come with a measuring device, so the child has to be directed to the visual cue for how much to add to the machine or dispenser. The timer helps the child know when he is to return to the laundry to continue his chore.

R. *Rely on Child's Learning Strength.* I found taking pictures of the child doing various chores and putting them into a scrapbook were helpful to support the child's memory and for the child to relate the chores to his actions. It helps them develop a personal identity as an individual capable of doing many things.

E. *Every Skill needs to Generalize.* Once the child can perform the laundry routine independently, you want to teach in a variety of environments because the details will be different. When we went on vacation, we did laundry at a public laundry, or hotel laundry, or in the vacation house. The first time we went to a laundry, I was surprised that David could not identify the washers and dryers because they looked different from the ones at home. In addition, one has to put money into the machines to run them. There may not be a soap dispenser, so the soap goes into the washing machine. If the soap and softener come in a different container, this may cause confusion for the child.

<u>S.</u> *Strive for Independence*. The goal is for the child to do his own laundry without supervision. If independence is lacking, consider additional structure to help the child, such as a visual chart.

<u>C.H.O.R.E.S. Bed making</u>

<u>C.</u> *Chart the Steps*. When you are ready to teach the more complex skill of making the bed, using an instruction chart can be helpful. This allows the task to be individualized to the child, provides information about the type of assistance the child requires and enables one to evaluate progress toward independence. If someone else is also teaching the skill, this chart is essential to keep the steps in sequence and track the changing supports needed. Children with autism focus on details and you are teaching to the details, such as giving visual cues for where covers touch on both sides of the bed.

<u>H.</u> *Have Success in Plan*. When David first started making the bed, I needed to make it as easy as possible, so he could do it independently. My neighbor, who also had a child with autism, suggested a comforter with a sheet cover that could be removed for washing. The comforter was not tucked at the bottom. To make his bed, I would take David's hands and grab the top of the comforter to pull it over the pillows. Very quickly he responded and could do this independently.

<u>O.</u> *Organize Materials and Simplify Instruction.* When verbalizing, speak slowly so the child can process language or use music to sing the instruction to him, or simply make the activity more fun. It is always important to praise effort and not just completion of the task. Don't worry if the bed isn't made perfectly, because independence is more important than perfection.

<u>R.</u> *Rely on Child's Learning Strengths*. One challenge, when putting on the bottom fitted sheet, is to get the sheet positioned properly on the bed with regards to width versus length. When David had difficulties finding the correct corner of the sheet, I put one of his hands on one corner and the other hand on the other corner of the width of the sheet and stretched it on the length of the bed, stating *"Oops, doesn't fit."* Then I moved his hands - still holding the sheet - to the width of the bed, so he could see that this is where the corners should be placed. I would sometimes sing, *"This is the way we make the bed, make the bed, make the bed. This is the way we make the bed, early in the morning."*

E. *Every Skill Needs to Generalize.* The task or chore is learned by rote, so when the bed is different or the linens are different, it requires further instruction. We had a travel trailer with a single bed for David. He had to learn to make this bed. Of course, it is usually much easier and faster than the initial training.

S. *Strive for Independence.* As the child is learning, he will make mistakes. Always give him time to correct the mistakes, but not so long as to frustrate him. You will notice that on the instruction chart that I started with hand-over-hand assistance. When he had difficulty getting the bottom sheet tucked under the mattress, I lifted the mattress slightly. After more experience, he was able to add this step. Parents are busy and it is always easier and faster to do it for the child, but this does not teach independence.

Bed Making Instruction Chart

Date: _____   Name: _____
I = Independent   PA = partial assistance
H/H = Hand over hand   T = Touch Assistance   V = verbal

Step	Assistance	Date	Change in Assistance
Take off sheets	I		
Put on bottom fitted sheet	H/H If corner of sheet doesn't stay, put your hands over his, grab the corner of sheet and pull it over the mattress		
Put on top flat sheet	PA – has difficulty getting sheet centered on bed, so doesn't drape over one side so shift his focus to spot (top of bedrail) where sheet should touch on each side of bed.		
Tuck sheet under mattress at bottom of bed	PA – may lift mattress slightly while he pushes sheet under mattress		
Put comforter on bed	PA – place his hand on spot (top of bedrail) where the side of comforter should touch.		

Chore Schedules

The daily and weekly chores are activities that one needs to do as an adult in order to live independently. The schedule avoids the organization and planning difficulties the child with autism experiences. It is really no different than many adults who make "to do" lists in order to remember what needs to be done. As I am now a senior citizen, I need more written lists, calendar schedules and routines to help me function. Each skill has to begin at an easy level that ensures success. When teaching children with autism, we are teaching to their strengths of attention to details and rote memory. In addition, written and/or picture schedules are used to support brain deficits with memory and sequencing behaviors.

The following are examples of chore schedules.

Example of a Daily Chore Schedule

Daily Chores	Sun.	Mon.	Tue.	Wed.	Thurs.	Fri.	Sat.	Sticker Reward
1. Empty Dishwasher								
2. Put dirty dishes into Dishwasher								
3. Shake rugs outside								
4. Swiffer floor; left to right; top to bottom								
5. Put rugs back on floor								
6. Take out trash								
7. Set the table								

Example of a Weekly Chore Schedule

Thursday Chores	Sticker for Completion
1. Remove bed linens for laundry	
2. Collect dirty linens, bath towels and washcloth, and dirty clothes from hamper and take to laundry room	
3. Vacuum bedroom (left to right; top to bottom)	
4. Dust bedroom	
5. Clean shower, sink, toilet	
6. Shake out rug, mop floor	
7. Do two loads of laundry – wash, dry, fold	
8. Make bed with clean linens; put clothes in dresser	

Teaching in Community Environments

The child with autism needs to be taught behaviors (routines/skills) in a variety of community environments. In this chapter I will provide a C.H.O.R.E.S. strategy for shopping in a grocery store, and eating in fast-food restaurants, cafeterias and sit-down restaurants.

In a grocery store, the child needs to learn how to push a cart through the store, locate items, put them into the basket, find a checkout, pay for items, locate the car, put items into the car and locate the area to return the cart. Since everything cannot be taught at once, it takes many years to build independence in these environments.

The sample instructional chart for grocery shopping has broken the process into steps, so you know what you are teaching and what assistance the child requires. Since teachers usually change every year and our children do not reveal their skills, it is important to have documentation. The chart should be adjusted to show what you are teaching and what supports are needed for each step. The chart also allows for updating the "Change in Assistance" column as he progresses.

SAMPLE INSTRUCTIONAL ACTIVITY – GROCERY SHOPPING

Name_____   I = Independent   PA = Partial Assist

STEP	ASSISTANCE	DATE	COMMENTS
1. Get Cart	Put child's hand on cart		
2. Put clipboard And list on cart	I		
3. Push Cart	PA		Difficulty predicting the Behavior of others. Hold Handle and if other people present are passing, teacher can stop cart and release cart when clear.
4. Locate food items	I		
5. Mark items off list	I		
6. Locate checkout, observe social cues for open lane	PA		Check to see that he identifies cues, such as light on, clerk at register, people in line, lane for limited items or open/closed sign. Careful or he will look to see where you are going as a clue.
7. Put purchases on conveyor belt	I		
8. Hand store card to clerk for store discounts	I		
9. Pay for purchase with credit card (or cash)	I		
10. Put bags into cart	I		
11. Push cart to car	PA		Observe closely that he crosses road safely
12. Load groceries into car	PA		May need assistance to lay items down that may slide while driving.
13. Put cart in corral	PA		Observe that he looks and crosses road safely

<u>C.</u> *Create an Instructional Chart.* An example is provided for you.

<u>H.</u> *Have Success in Plan.* The first goal is to establish the structure with a clear beginning and ending with the grocery cart. I found it best to train in the environment when it is quiet, so there will be fewer distractions. The first basic goal is to teach the child to hold onto the handle of a shopping cart with you standing behind the child. I started by putting my hands over his hands to ensure he would not run away. This provides a boundary and indicates what the child should do in this environment.

If we are going to make the process successful for the child, then we need to incorporate what he knows. Most children with autism eat the same things, so when we go into the grocery store, they should have a list (pictures, words, or box labels) of the foods they eat. When you locate an item, physically put the child's hand on the list indicating the item and then move the child toward the item for him to pick it up and place it in the cart. As the child begins to understand and respond, you can add steps that you think the child is ready to master. By putting the steps together and teaching it every week, the child learns a complete routine for functioning in the grocery store.

<u>O.</u> *Organize Materials and Simplify Instruction.* The child needs a list of items to buy. Most children with autism eat the same things, so when we go into the grocery store, they should have a list (pictures, words, or box labels) of the foods they eat. I used the list on a clipboard with a colored pencil attached. When you locate an item, physically put the child's hand on the list indicating the item and then move the child toward the item for him to pick it up and place it in the cart. He can then mark the item on the list with the pencil.

Although the chart includes a complete routine, you start with only the basic structure to give the child an opportunity to adapt. To get started, say to the child, *"Time to buy food. We get a cart first."* Put the child's hands on the handle of the cart to show him what he does in this environment. It also prevents him from running away.

When you come to something the child eats, tell him *"Cereal"*, and physically guide him through the motions of picking up the box and putting it into the basket. Then put his hands back onto the handle of the cart. You want to keep the child participating in the process as much as possible. When you get to the checkout, the child should help put groceries on the conveyor belt. He should help get the groceries into the car and put the cart away.

Once the child is comfortable in the environment, there is opportunity to teach details about where items are located, and the different ways foods can be packaged. It is always best to use something of interest to the child and to teach from the child's perspective.

David ate tater tots for breakfast, so I made a list of different ways potatoes are sold, such as fresh, frozen, boxed, canned, and prepared. Prior to going to the store, I showed him the list and told him we would locate potatoes in different areas of the store. He could check them off as we found them. We often assume as we go through a grocery store that the child can "see" the different types of foods, but a child with autism does not observe and imitate so he needs to be taught everything.

<u>R.</u> *Rely on Child's Learning Strengths.* We always try to create visuals to assist the child in understanding what he is buying and include the foods he likes. Initially, I created a list with box or can labels taped to the paper. Later, I was able to simply write the item on the paper and eventually, he was able to make the list. David liked to repeat some food commercials, such as Hellman's mayonnaise and Cool Whip. I put the items on the grocery list, so David could learn to locate them in the store. Because the items had meaning for him, he was very excited.

<u>E.</u> *Every Skill needs to Generalize.* Every grocery store is a little different, from the location of items, the type of items stocked, and the variety of social cues for checkout lanes. Since the child with autism attends to details, you have to teach to the details. This requires training in a variety of stores. Shopping carts are available in most stores, so the use of the cart can be generalized to many environments. This is advantageous for anyone who has a child who tends to run away in public places. By helping the child understand the purpose of being in an environment and what he does in that environment, it reduces the unwanted behaviors.

<u>S.</u> *Strive for Independence.* The goal is always for the child to do a task himself and we provide the necessary steps and supports to achieve that goal.

Teaching and Evaluating

You can't teach everything at once, so you have to decide what you are teaching and why you are teaching it. If the situation becomes stressful for the child, then learning will not occur. You want to look for teaching opportunities that incorporate something that is meaningful for the child. For example, if the child eats fruit, you can show him the different types of fruit. He can touch it, smell it, and take some home to taste it. David became fascinated with all the different types of pears and he had to try all of them.

When the basic routine is learned, additional instruction is needed, such as: 1) locate new items; 2) identify areas of the store for fresh fruit and vegetables, frozen food, canned foods, boxed foods, meat department, refrigerated items; 3) How to ask for assistance; 4) How to pay for items – cash, credit or debit card.

Prior to the day's training, show the child the clipboard that indicates what he is going to do that day. For example, if you are going to have him identify various forms of food, use pictures to assist the child's memory and he can check the items off as he locates them.

One of the most difficult tasks for the child is locating the checkout. There are various social cues to attend to and they can vary by store. Some checkout lanes are express and allow only a few items. Some checkout lanes have lights or signs to indicate they are open. One of the most obvious signs to most people is a person working the checkout, but sometimes the person is in training or closing a register and it is not actually open for business. We make these inferences quickly and easily, but the child with autism doesn't have the long-distance connections to understand meaning of these various social cues.

Another challenge for the child with autism will be pushing the cart through the store. The child has to consider the location of other people and how to get around people. The difficulties with this skill include knowing what to focus on and interpreting the behavior of others. I started the training with me actually controlling the cart and David holding onto the handle. If the store is crowded, he may have to stop and wait for the aisle to clear. Since you can't be teaching two things at once, I recommend teaching the child to push the cart when it is a quiet time at the store and he is buying

194

items very familiar to him. Don't expect him to rapidly switch attention between pushing the cart and locating items to buy.

Evaluation of progress is easy. You can stand back and watch the child independently shop in the store. If there are problem areas, then they are easily identified. One of the first times I closely observed David to evaluate his progress, I discovered he was looking at my feet to determine where to push the grocery cart. If I turned my foot to the right, he went right; if I turned my foot to the left, he went left.

C.H.O.R.E.S. Fast-Food Restaurants

Children with autism need to learn to function in a variety of restaurant situations, including fast food, sit-down, and cafeteria. Each one is different and the child needs to learn the behaviors for each one. Although it seems like a lot of work, it is worth it. As an adult, my son easily functions in these environments and enjoys a variety of foods.

SAMPLE INSTRUCTIONAL CHART – FAST FOOD
Name_____   I =Independent   PA = Partial Assist
N/A = Not Teaching this step

STEP	ASSISTANCE	DATE	COMMENTS
1. Locate order line	PA		Difficulty staying in line and understanding boundaries – stand next to child and physically prompt if needed.
2. Read order	PA		How to order depends on child's skill. Some can read order, order by number or verbalize.
3. Pay for order	N/A		
4. Take tray to table	I		
5. Take cup to beverage station/fill with ice and choice of drink	I		
6. Take trash to trash can	I		

C. *Chart the Details*. A sample instructional chart is included. In a fast-food restaurant, you start with a simple routine to allow the child to become comfortable in the environment.

H. *Have Success in the Plan.* I found teaching in fast-food restaurants more difficult than cafeterias or sit-down restaurants. It requires waiting in lines. I would try to find times that were very quiet, so we did not have to wait in line.

O. *Organize Materials and Simplify Instruction*. In the beginning, I would have him stand at the counter and put his hands on the counter (so he could not run away). It can be helpful to have him hold a napkin or utensil to remember that it is time to eat. He had to carry his tray from the counter to a table. At first, I would carry the drinks separately as he was less likely to spill it. Most fast food places now provide machines for customers to obtain their own drinks. When he finished eating, he would carry his tray to the trashcan, empty the trash and put his tray in the specified area. He may need to be physically guided through the actions in the beginning. Remember, you are not teaching language and you don't want him to rely on you telling him what to do.

R. *Rely on Child's Learning Strengths*. Ordering food is a major step for the child and requires a consideration of each child's strengths. David loves numbers and in some places the food items are numbered. When he was first starting, he always ate the same thing, so I could provide a picture with the words on a piece of paper. Since he found eye contact distracting, he could look at the paper to say what he wanted. If the clerk did not understand, David did not want to repeat his order, and I often had to intervene. If he had stated his order, I considered it a success and repeated the order for him. Even though our children may be older when learning to function in the community, we need to remember to support their efforts in the beginning to give them time to adjust. We need to praise effort, not perfection, and make the experience successful.

E. *Every Skill needs to Generalize.* One day, after eating in a restaurant, my five-year old could not locate the trashcan. Looking for differences in the situation, it became apparent we had been going to McDonald's where the trashcan had a symbol on it. This restaurant lacked the symbol. Since children with autism focus on differences, he could not locate the trashcan without the symbol. This is another example of lack of generalization that you will encounter when working with a child with autism.

When a lack of generalization occurs, we have to teach the child to manage the behavior in a variety of environments. First, we have to recognize the differences, as trash containers can be large or small, open or closed, with different colors and shapes. I would help David to identify and use the different types of trash containers in various environments.

<u>S</u>. *Strive for Independence*. The goal is independence so every teaching strategy is an attempt to support and increase the child's ability to do the task on his own. Repeating the routines enables the child to use his strength of rote memory and attention to details.

C.H.O.R.E.S. Cafeteria

SAMPLE INSTRUCTIONAL CHART - CAFETERIA
Name ⎯⎯⎯   I =Independence   PA = Partial Assist

STEP	ASSISTANCE	DATE	COMMENTS
1. Review food items, visually or chart.	PA		Assist with choices before the line by noting foods student likes. Direct (tap wall or move child's hand) attention to food list to make choices, of view food, if possible.
2. Get tray and silverware	I		Student has some difficulty following line so teacher can hold his tray to prevent child moving it forward, if needed.
3. Attend to first server, respond with choice or "No thank you."	PA		Difficulty shifting attention to various servers and knowing who is speaking to him. Can tell child the server will look at him when it is his turn. If difficulty processing server's voice, repeat message.
4. Put items on tray when given by server	I		
5. Attend to entrée server, respond with choice	PA		At first, David pointed to his choice and I stated it to the server. Later, he was able to verbalize choice.
6. Attend to	PA		

next server, respond with choice			
7. Dessert, if wanted	I		
9. Attend to bread server, respond with choice or "No thank you."	PA		
120. Attend to drink server, respond with choice	PA		
14. End of line, take bill.	I		
15. Take tray. Locate table	I		
16. Get in line to pay with money ready	PA		Standing in line can be difficult. Wait until only one person in line if possible.
17. Pay for food	PA		Individualize to skills of child. If pay with cash, have money ready. Can use charge card if student signs name.

<u>C</u>. *Chart the Details.* In a cafeteria, there is a line of people. You have to pick up a tray and silverware, move along the line and attend to multiple food servers. At the end of the line, you either pay or pick up a receipt in order to pay when you exit. In most cafeterias, someone clears the table, but some have an area for the customer to leave his tray and dishes. A sample instructional chart is included.

<u>H</u>. *Have Success in Plan.* Most children with autism have limited food choices. David would eat meat with cheese, so I told him he would have this for lunch at the cafeteria. This is not the time to expand food choices because the training is focused on proper behavior in this environment. At first, I would have him in front of me and put the tray and silverware in front of him. When we came to his entrée, I told him "Look, there is your cheeseburger." David was familiar with carrying his tray to the table, so this step was not difficult. Once the child becomes more comfortable in this environment, then you can add steps.

<u>O.</u> **Organize Materials and Simplify Instruction.** Training in a cafeteria was easier in some ways, because the child can see the food and make choices before entering the line. Keep it simply at first by providing more support for the child, such as having him point to what he wants, while you tell the server. With several food servers, the student may be confused as to who is speaking to him. Once he is more comfortable in the environment, it may be helpful to indicate the serve will look at him when it is his turn to order.

<u>R.</u> **Rely on Child's Learning Strengths.** Cafeterias as great because so much is visible and he does not have to rely on memory. In addition, the child can point to what he wants.

<u>E.</u> **Every Skill needs to Generalize.** Once the child can manage in one cafeteria, it is helpful to find other cafeterias for him to practice his skills. Each one is a little different and will serve different items, so he has to have time to adjust to the differences.

<u>S.</u> *Strive for Independence.* If payment is required at the end of the cafeteria line, then this was the most difficult for David to handle, because he didn't have time to prepare himself. He would be slow getting his money ready and this would cause impatience in people in the line. Therefore, you have to make a judgment of when it is time to add this step and how to make it efficient and successful. I would have David hold a bill on his tray ready to pay for the end of the line and show him how to put the change on his tray until he got to the table. There were other cafeterias where one paid on the way out and this was easier to teach David to look at the bill and count his money to pay the bill prior to getting into the line.

C.H.O.R.E.S. Sit-down Restaurant

<u>C.</u> *Chart the Details.* A sample instructional chart is included. With a sit-down restaurant, you are usually greeted with a host, but sometimes there is a sign to seat yourself. Once seated, someone usually asks you what you want to drink. After bringing drinks, you usually order your food and then wait for the food to be delivered.

<u>H.</u> *Have Success in the Plan.* The first visits will focus on waiting at the table and proper eating behavior. The child should already know how to eat properly at home, so this is generalizing his skill. The instructional charts are designed for the teacher to use with a child who is comfortable in the

environment with the basic routine. You will not be teaching all steps at one time, as you do not want to overwhelm the child. For example, determining the tip and paying the bill will only be possible when the child has some math skills. David has a chart he carries in his wallet to determine the amount for a tip.

<u>O</u>. *Organize Materials and Simplify Instruction.* The waiting time for the food to be delivered can be difficult so I would bring David a hand-held game to play. In addition, you can order an appetizer that might shorten the waiting time.

<u>R</u>. *Rely on the Child's Learning Strengths.* The sit-down restaurant is one situation where the inability to recognize faces can be a challenge for a person with autism. On several occasions, David would make a service request to the wrong server, because he could not recognize the person who was serving us. If the server wears a nametag, it is helpful. Otherwise, we would help him identify the server.

<u>E</u>. *Every Skill needs to Generalize.* Every restaurant is a little different and the child needs to experience these differences. The more practice he has, the stronger the rote memory skills become.

S. *Strive for Independence.* The instructional charts are helpful to maintain a focus on what needs to be taught toward the goal of adult independence. It is easy to get into a routine and fail to continue the instruction needed for the child. These charts are educational plans that need to be reviewed every year to determine what steps need to be addressed.

When we started going to restaurants, David would always order his cheeseburger and fries. Once we taught him the parts of the menu and how one can order "sides" with an entrée, he soon started ordering different things. Of course, we were also teaching him in a grocery store and he was learning to cook, so his food choices expanded. As an adult, he is very proficient at placing his order and enjoying a wide variety of foods.

SAMPLE INSTRUCTIONAL CHART: SIT-DOWN RESTAURANT

Name_____   I = Independent   PA = Partial Assist

STEP	ASSISTANCE	DATE	COMMENTS
1. Respond to host with number in party	PA		Prepare child prior to entering restaurant.
2. Respond to server with drink order	PA		Ensure child is given time to review drinking options on the menu.
3. Review menu and make choices	PA		Review items child likes on the menu.
4. Respond to server by pointing to choices or verbalizing choices	PA		If child uses low voice, you may have to repeat it. Instruct child to turn face toward server when making order.
5. Plan for waiting behavior – can play hand-held game	PA		Bring book or game to help with waiting behavior
6. Respond politely with "thank you" when food is served or drink refilled	PA		
7. Politely ask server for any needed items	PA		Tell child when the server comes to the table, he can say "water please" and later extend to 'Please bring me some water when you get a chance" If necessary, write it down and he can read it.
8. Demonstrates proper eating behavior			Instruct as needed
9. Review bill, determine tip, and pay bill	Last step to add to routine		

Conclusion

The long-term goal is independent adult functioning and the short-term goals are teaching routines that will enable the child to reach that long-term goal. Although you will not teach all the routines at one time, it is helpful to prepare charts, so you won't forget to stay on track for teaching. The child needs to learn what behaviors are expected in every environment.

Although it seems like a great deal of work, I can assure you the results are worth it. My son is independent with self-care, chores, shopping in the grocery store and eating in restaurants. He likes to cook and we enjoy his cookies, cakes, and casseroles. We can take him to the best restaurants and be assured that he knows how to order and behave properly.

He cuts the grass, uses a blower to clean debris from the driveway, helps dig holes for planting, and spreads mulch. People often think he is "high functioning" and are unaware of his dependence on rote memory and routines. He cannot carry on a conversation, but he can use language to meet his needs and function in our society.

Summary of Teaching Strategies

1. Children with autism are unable to handle unique or novel situations, because they do not have associative memories that can be retrieved and built upon, and they don't observe and imitate. Therefore, they must be taught routines in many different environments. Once the child becomes comfortable in an environment, then he is able to handle changes and more steps in the routine.

2. Teaching strategies should try to incorporate the interests of the child, such as buying items in the grocery store that the child likes, as opposed to what a parent would like the child to eat.

3. Many chores can be structured with the simple instruction of left to right; top to bottom, such as washing windows, washing a car, vacuuming or sweeping floors.

4. Teaching chores increases the child's ability to function more independently and self-reliantly as an adult. It may make the difference between being able to live in their own apartment with supports, rather than a group home that tends to rely on adult verbal instruction for daily activities.

5. If the child has unwanted behaviors, review your teaching strategies and provide more support.

Chapter 12

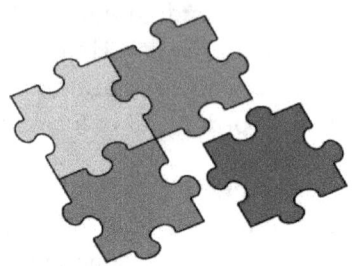

Teaching Recreation, Job-Skills, and Social Skills
Learning is not the result of teaching to know. Learning is the result of doing. Cheryl Merritt.

Most children naturally run and play. They learn to ride bikes and play team sports, but our children with autism are often happy in a room repeating an activity over and over. They get very little exercise. Exercise is extremely important for everyone. Therefore, physical exercise should be included in the child's schedule and specifically taught. Exercise can be structured with counting, such as jumping on a small trampoline while counting to 100, or counting jumps into the pool.

Temple Grandin has been telling us (2008, **The Way I See It**) that children with autism benefit greatly by exercise and this is supported by research. John Medina devotes an entire chapter in his book, **Brain Rules** (2008), on the benefits of exercise, based on neurological research.

Jennifer McIlwee Myers in her book (2010) **How to Teach Life Skills to Kids with Autism or Asperger's,** writes that active group activities (team sports) is NOT the "exercise" we are referring to for children with autism, but rather activities that provide sustained effort to support strong muscles and brain health, such as jumping, running, swimming, and gymnastics. Mrs. Myers also notes that some people with autism may prefer to exercise in non-public situations. I found private lessons were a good start to establish the skill, and then I transferred the exercise to a public place or team, where social skills must be taught.

We often make the mistake of assuming that when the person with autism gets older and he can do more, he will be able to learn like his nondisabled peers. I discovered that the brain deficits are not cured and will continue to require accommodations.

Transition instruction into adulthood needs to include activities one can use as an adult. An adult needs exercise, recreation activities, and job skills. David participates in community activities for exercise, such as water aerobics, recreational activities in the community, such as bingo and board games. He also enjoys going to movies, stage productions, and restaurants.

During David's teenage years, he received individual lessons in art, gymnastics, and swimming. Individual lessons are important, because the child's brain can't process what is important to focus on and what is irrelevant to the activity. This is where the concept of teaching one thing at a time becomes meaningful. You are not teaching language or social skills in these individual lessons.

When the skill is learned and it is time to transfer the skill to a group setting, the focus of teaching changes. The presence of more people requires some basic social skills, such as waiting your turn or walking in line or basic greetings and communication. The group settings we used were community art classes, a gymnastics competitive team, and Special Olympics swimming. The following is a review of teaching each skill with the strategies used. These are not theoretical textbook examples, but real-life experiences including situations that can occur during the teaching process.

Gymnastics

David started taking private gymnastic lessons at the age of twelve. Terri was a very experienced coach. When David had difficulty observing and imitating, she guided his body through the motions, so he could get the feel of it. For example, on the trampoline, she physically flipped his body, so he would get the feel of it. Once he could make flips in gymnastics, he easily learned to flip in swimming, at the end of the lane, while doing laps.

Terri taught David as if he were blind and/or deaf. When she spoke to him, she put her hands in her pockets, so she would not gesture while talking. She realized David had difficulty knowing what to focus on, so this reduced his brain processing challenges. If she gestured or demonstrated something, she would not speak.

After learning a few skills, David started dropping to the floor and did not want to work anymore. You can never interpret behavior as if he were a typically developing child. When the skill training does not go well, we need to look at changing our teaching strategies, and not blame the child. It is better to assume that he doesn't understand the situation, and you need to provide more structure. It was time to add visuals.

I brought a clipboard with written lessons on it, consisting of the name of each skill and how many were to be performed. David would mark the chart for completion after each skill. This had an immediate impact on his behavior, for he understood what was expected and that there was a beginning and ending. As a "reward" for completion of his lesson, he wanted to climb the hanging rope. This was not something I would have thought would be rewarding to him, as it is used for training muscle strength, but we have to remember that children with autism have a different perspective.

In gymnastics, once basic skills are learned, they are put together into routines. There is a standard routine for an entry-level gymnast for each event: floor, high-bar, pommel horse, parallel bars and vault. This was perfect for David's rote-memory learning style, because every routine is taught the same way over and over, until he no longer has to think about it.

Terri gave me a videotape of the routines and David watched them at home. You might wonder how he could learn from it, if he doesn't observe and imitate. The videotape will remain the same each time he views it, and it doesn't require any judgment as to where to focus, and there are no distractions (no talking). Since David could already perform the skills, viewing the film should stimulate the motor neurons that he would use performing the skill himself, and this teaches to rote memory.

When David was learning the floor routine, we encountered a problem. When he stands and does nothing, we know he doesn't understand something. David uses objects very well, but this was an open space. Although there are clear boundaries around the floor mat, there is no visual guidance, when the child is performing from one corner of the floor to another. We added ropes to create a visual boundary from one corner to the other, so David knew he was to perform within that area. After a few times, we were able to remove the rope and he could perform.

After a year of private lessons, Terri suggested David might be able to handle an entry-level competitive team. At the gym, there were three entry-level teams. The athletes were five years younger than David, but he didn't seem to notice or care that he towered above them. Sometimes professionals and parents worry too much about something being age-appropriate, when it isn't a problem for the child with autism.

Terri picked a team that had a boy's coach she thought would work well with David. We decided the new coach, Domingo, should work with David during the individual (private) lessons. David had a few lessons with Domingo prior to starting on the team, so Terri could share her teaching strategies and David's skill level.

During the individual lessons, Domingo would try to improve David's skills within each routine. After performing a routine, the coach would try to provide a verbal correction, such as *"Point your toes"*. David responded, *"I did"* and he became increasingly agitated with each correction. Whenever there is a problem with the child's behavior, we must first consider what we may have done wrong, before we can provide more support for the child.

In order for David to understand the criticism, he would have to imagine himself performing the skill, by remembering what he had just done. But children with autism have associative memory difficulties and can't imagine what they have done. David could perform the skill from rote memory, but could not imagine his performance.

I brought a video camera to the next lesson and filmed David performing his skills. When the coach wanted to make a correction, I would rewind the tape. They would look at the monitor of the camera, so David had a visual picture of the imperfections to be corrected. This solved the problem because David did not have to rely on his impaired memory. David could not tell us what the problem was and it is up to others to understand and support learning deficits.

The next challenge was having David join the team during practice sessions. The gym would be filled with children. We were all a little concerned about how David would react, because the private lessons occurred when it was less crowded in the gym. The entire staff at the center had a meeting and worked together to make this successful. The first time David participated in the team practice, the entire coaching staff was in the gym and they created extra space between David's team and the other activities occurring in the gym. I sat with parents viewing through a glass wall.

After several group lessons, David's verbalizations started interfering with his functioning on the team. Because of the waiting time before David's turn to perform a routine, David would resort to repetitive behaviors, such as making sounds and talking to himself and finger flicking. I created a behavior contract with David that described appropriate behavior (sit quietly with hands in your lap; watch your teammate perform). If he demonstrated appropriate behavior during the team practice, he could climb the ropes at the end of the lesson. Much to my relief, the contract was effective and he could continue on the team. We often forget that we have to teach children with autim "waiting behavior", because we don't teach that to typical children. You have to be specific about what behavior is expected in every situation.

During one team lesson, Coach Domingo solved a baffling problem. They were practicing their floor routines and several boys had completed the routine, and now it was David's turn. The coach directed him to a starting corner. David stood there, and he did not start his routine. What could be the problem? The coach directed him to another corner of the floor, and David performed beautifully.

The coach realized that during the individual lessons, David had done the floor routine from only one corner, so he perceived the other corners as different. This is a perfect example of the lack of generalization that is so difficult for children with autism. During the next individual lesson, David was taught to perform the floor routine from each corner. If we don't understand how the child thinks and learns, we may interpret behavior as willfully defiant or lacking motivation. Rather than blame the child, we must look for alternative ways to support the child's learning style.

Shortly before the first competition, Domingo and I spent some private lesson time to prepare David for what to expect. He practices walking from one area to another, and saluting to the judges before each performance. One of his mistakes during practice was saluting without facing the judge. Facing the judge is a social skill that has to be specifically taught.

During the first competition, we learned that we had forgotten one other accommodation. When he started his high bar routine, he dropped to the floor twice. What was the problem? He announced that he had to go to the bathroom – we had forgotten to program a toilet break!

David participated in several competitions and won some awards. We never discussed his performance scores, because for our purposes, competition was not important: it was successful participation that was the goal for David. Because children with autism focus on details, one has to be careful when teaching about scores in competitive games. I have observed children with autism focusing on their scores, and getting very upset about them. We need to help our children focus on what is important about games and that is the social participation.

Life is full of changes and eventually we had to change coaches. Unfortunately, this new coach could not believe David could do gymnastics. I showed him videotapes, but soon realized the low expectations from this person would interfere with progress, and could possibly affect David's behaviors. It was time to move on. It had been a successful experience, so David's self-esteem received a boost and he gained body strength and coordination.

Typical children can imagine themselves in the future. They would observe the older gymnasts who were attempting to win scholarships for college or prepare for the Olympics and some would create these goals for themselves. Associational memories enable one to connect the past to the future. The child with autism will not associate the skills with future goals or other meanings – such as performance on a team, working for trophies or building a skill that enables one to earn scholarships for school.

Typical children, who are learning gymnastics or cheerleading, will perform skills in various areas, such as the yard, or the beach. David never tried to do any skills elsewhere, because he associated gymnastics with the place he learned. Without the ability to generalize skills to other areas, David never seemed to care that we stopped gymnastics. We just moved on to other activities.

Swimming

At age thirteen, David started private swimming lessons during the summer at our neighborhood pool. His teacher was excellent at helping him get the feel of the strokes. He responded quickly and learned several different swim strokes, but he only used the strokes during the swim lessons. Just like gymnastics, he would not generalize the learning from the training class to another time or situation.

The next summer, David started swim lessons again with the same person. This time, David was assigned homework, where he would swim a specified number of laps, using the different strokes. It was structured with numbers, so he did four lengths of freestyle stroke, four lengths of backstroke, four lengths of breaststroke and four lengths of his choice (4-4-4-4). By the end of the summer, we increased it to 8-4-4-4.

At age seventeen, David joined a Special Olympics swim team. Once again, when becoming part of a group, the teaching changes focus to group adjustment. Whenever David started with a group situation, I noticed a drop in his skills, probably because of the stress of the new situation. Once he adjusts to the group, his skill levels return to normal.

Jerry and I attended the practice sessions, so David had the supports needed to ensure success. One of the lessons for David was to change his clothes independently in the men's locker room. This proved to be the most important lesson, because as an adult, he now attends a water aerobics class independently.

There were two special education teachers for this team. We were very disappointed that they didn't provide much instruction or enthusiasm. Fortunately, we had a neighbor, David Koehn, who was a competitive high school swimmer, and he volunteered to provide private instructions. This experience was quite beneficial as David's skills increased tremendously, and he had experience interacting with someone near his own age.

At the end of the year, it was time to go to Omaha, Nebraska for the State Special Olympics event. All the participants were gathered together on the floor of a gymnasium located next to the pool. Teams were sitting on blankets on the floor with the coaches. When it was time for the team to swim, they formed a line and left the area to go to the pool. Unfortunately, David Koehn was unable to attend, so I stayed with David and Jerry sat with parents observing the event.

I ran to the observation area to watch and then returned to the waiting area. Much to my surprise, after completing the event, everyone returned to the blanket where the coaches were sitting, except David.

Teachers naturally assume a seventeen year old will stay with the group, but in this crowded situation, David was distracted, and unable to focus on staying with the group. I wandered around the room looking for David, and finally located him. I guided him back to his group.

David enjoyed the event and he was very successful. He came in first place for the breaststroke. He was the only child to do a flip turn and the parents watching broke out in cheers, when they saw this. In addition, David was not allowed to start on the side of the pool and dive into the water. Everyone was required to get into the water and start from a standing position. I don't understand why there is such low expectations for children with disabilities. I know it is a challenge to teach children with disabilities and many don't want to take the time or don't know how to teach.

As an adult, David goes to water aerobics classes twice a week with a group of senior citizens (mainly women). Often educators become overly concerned about "age appropriate" activities, and this can restrict opportunities for people with autism. David is not concerned – as he seems unaware – that the rest of the group is elderly. He has done this for nine years and the women seem to enjoy his youthful enthusiasm. They sometimes have potlucks, and David looks forward to these and enjoys them. He is expected to make a dish to contribute. He is an accepted part of the group, but doesn't have social conversations.

Job Skills

Cutting the Grass

At age eight, David started cutting the grass by simply walking around the yard with his father, while holding onto the handle of the lawnmower. This was similar to learning to walk around the store, holding onto the handle of a grocery or shopping cart.

At age eleven, we decided it was time for him to learn to do the job independently. I created boundaries by cutting a rectangle and then demonstrated the difference between the cut grass and the tall grass by putting his hand on both. Once he could cut the grass within the rectangle, we extended it to cutting grass marked off by the flowerbeds, that were surrounded with black plastic edging.

The next summer, we encountered a problem. Fortunately, I was in the yard near him and heard a strange noise from the mower. The mower has a lever to engage the blade and David ignored the noise and started to engage the blade. I told him to *"Stop"!* The blade had been recently sharpened and apparently was not reattached tightly, so it was falling off.

Responding to novel situations are processed by long-distance connections in the brain, that are often deficient in autism. Once a routine is taught, there will always be new situations that need to be addressed.

One day, David was cutting the grass, when I saw him standing motionless in the yard. There was a hammock, hanging in front of him, blocking his path. Apparently, Jerry usually removed the hammock, but he was out of town. I watched him for a moment and when he didn't move, I intervened. Typically, the brain processes meaning to a situation to enable one to create a plan of action. With autism, everything is learned by routine and the ability to make judgments or to deal with novel situations requires associational memory, a deficit in autism.

Washing a Car

Because of David's lack of planning and organization skills, I gathered supplies for the task and put them all in a bucket, but that was the only thing I did right. For some unknown reason, I slipped back into the talk mode and tried to talk David through the job. I started by telling him to *"Wash the roof"* and *"Wash the hood."* I slowly realized, I was not teaching language and he would be dependent on me to direct him how to wash the car. He also seemed to think he only had to wash dirt that he could see. I then returned to a basic simple instruction of washing and rinsing from left to right and top to bottom.

Volunteer Work

When David was sixteen, he started volunteer work at a rehabilitation hospital for two afternoons per week. I was his job coach. His job was to clean tables in the cafeteria toward the end of the lunchtime, restock drinks and chips, and vacuum the floor. Since we know the child with autism has difficulty with planning and organization, then we have to support this problem. We don't want the person with autism to rely on someone telling him what to do, so he needs a visual chart or checklist to support his memory until the job becomes routine.

To prepare for his restocking chips and drinks, I prepared a checklist on a clipboard. This allowed him to mark how many drinks he needed to replace (mainly soft drinks and cartons of different types of milk). Once he completed the checklist, he went to the stock room, got a cart, put the soft drinks onto the cart, and then he went to the refrigeration unit to put the milk cartons onto the cart. He returned to the cafeteria to restock the items from his cart. To restock the chips, he rolled the display to the stockroom to the boxes of chips. He could refill the display using the basic guidance of left to right; top to bottom. When finished, the display was rolled back to its place in the cafeteria. The staff found the checklist for restocking drinks very convenient, and they started using it.

In the beginning, it helps to have a visual guide for the jobs to be completed. David was able to read, so it was easy for me to prepare a list of the items he needed. In preparation for cleaning tables, he needed a cloth, bucket, liquid cleaner, and water. Fortunately, the cleaner came from an automatic dispenser, so he didn't have to judge how much cleaner to put into the bucket. When cleaning tables, he dipped his cloth into the bucket, wrung it out and cleaned from left to right; top to bottom. He also wiped the seats clean in the same manner then pushed the seats under the table.

To vacuum, he had to locate the machine, take it to the eating area, and find the electrical outlet to connect the vacuum. Although he uses a vacuum at home, this was a much larger area, so he needed some visual cues to work one area at a time. When he started, he was unaware that if people were around, they could trip on the cord. I watched out for this, while he became accustomed to his job. Later, I directed his attention to people walking over the cord, and instructed him to wait for them and not pull on the cord as it might trip them. Once again, the person with autism has difficulty putting meaning to what he sees, so seeing people walking over the vacuum cord would not automatically indicate to him to be careful not to trip them.

The basic routine was learned easily and did not present many difficulties. The greatest challenge for David to function in this environment was learning proper social behavior. Sometimes people in the cafeteria would try to ask David a question and he would ignore them. I instructed David to say, "*I don't know*," because I thought this would be more acceptable than to ignore people. Initially, staff members would try to ask him to do something, without realizing that he was only able to follow a set routine. Once they understood the condition, we could add another chore to his routine, if needed.

David had to be taught specific behaviors, such as reporting to his boss when he arrived and when he was leaving, and to report when there was a problem, such as the vacuum didn't work. In addition, David needed instruction on what to do after completing work. I decided he could get a drink and/or a snack, pay for it and sit at a table. This was his reward after work.

One evening, David attended a social event at the hospital and sat next to a pleasant young lady. The next day, while David was working, this lady came into the cafeteria and was excited to speak to him. Unfortunately, she was unaware that David does not recognize faces, and would not remember her from the previous evening. He became frightened and ran to hide behind his boss. He identified his boss, because she wore a nametag, and he knew where she would be.

The first year consisted of direct teaching and supervision, but the second year, I did volunteer work in another area of the hospital. I was still available, but if David was to achieve independence, he needed to know he could do it.

One day, his boss had an interesting story to tell. There was a bathroom for staff off the kitchen area where she was washing her hands. David came in and used the toilet! Fortunately, she had teenagers herself, so she merely walked out and closed the door.

When I tried to explain to David that he was not to go into the bathroom if someone else was in there, he said, "*She wasn't using the toilet*". I told him she should have shut the door, so he would know the bathroom was occupied, but in the future, he was not to enter the bathroom if anyone was in there, even if they were only washing their hands or had forgotten to close the door. Social skills need to be specifically taught.

Social Skills

Every year, David participates in a bowling league with adults with disabilities. Most of the participants come bounding into the building enthusiastically greeting their friends. They look for where they are to bowl based on the location of their teammates. They often have a difficult time focusing on bowling, because they are too busy talking and socializing. For these participants, the social interaction with friends is more important than the bowling.

In the midst of the chaos, there are a few with autism who have also looked forward to bowling and being with their friends, but they quietly stride into the building, locate their names on the screen above each alley to indicate where they go, sit down, and put on their bowling shoes. They concentrate on the game and are often focused on their scores, rarely interacting with their friends. They can spend an entire evening next to their friend on the team and only give a quick "hello" or a "high five," but they know one another and enjoy bowling together.

Although these are two very different social styles, they work for the individuals. Many parents spend years hoping their child with autism will have friends to talk, play and "hang-out" with. We have to be careful about imposing our personal ideas or needs onto our children. For those with autism, it isn't about the social interaction with friends as much as functioning in a social environment around other people. As Temple Grandin tells us, we worry too much about the social interaction of children with autism and we need to teach skills that enable the child to be in a social environment with others, even if they can't carry on a social conversation.

Summary of Teaching Strategies

1. Children with autism learn a skill best with one-to-one instruction and then transfer the skill to a group, where the teaching strategy changes to accommodate social behavior. Teaching strategies may include helping the child get the feel of a motion or movement, such as doing a flip on a trampoline.

2. Numerous examples in this chapter reveal the brain differences in autism will continue to require some accommodations, even as the child becomes a teenager and young adult. After several gymnastics lessons, David

(a teenager) dropped to the floor and this was understood to be a lack of understanding of what was expected and not defiant behavior. When more structure was provided, then he easily followed the lessons. The lack of generalization was seen in the floor gymnastics routine, when David was only able to perform the routine from one corner, then had to be specifically taught from all four corners. A video recorder was used in gymnastics lessons to assist his associative memory: imaging himself doing something. The recording enabled David to see his performance, while the coach made suggestions to improve.

3. Transition training to adulthood needs to include activities for exercise, recreation (board games, bingo), and hobbies (beading, weaving, art), useful to the individual as an adult. After the skill is taught, it is transferred to a group situation to include real-life experiences in social behavior.

4. Exercise that produces sustained effort, such as running, jumping, swimming or gymnastics, is important for children with autism. This does not include team sports (such as basketball, baseball and football) that can stress a child because it demands too much social interaction and social knowledge. Team sports that rely on individual performance (such as bowling, golf, and gymnastics) are better options for individuals with autism.

5. Teaching manners and kindness to others are more important than trying to teach how to make eye contact, have a conversation or ask questions.

6. Self-care skills, hobbies and work skills, and recreation for exercise, enable individuals with autism to have more independence, self-reliance, and a better quality of life. This also creates more opportunities for living arrangements, when the person does not require a great deal of supervision or assistance with activities of daily living.

A.P.P.R.E.C.I.A.T.E. THE CHILD WITH AUTISM
(A Behavior Management Program)
Cheryl S. Merritt

A. Accept the Child. The first step in developing a behavior management program for a child with autism is to view the child as wonderful and capable so he can live up to our expectations. The power of expectation is tremendous. If we view a child's behavior as bizarre simply because he has the label of autism, we will not be able to see the communicative intent of the behavior. We all have behaviors in private that we suppress when someone walks into the room. We often forget that children with autism do not suppress behaviors to conform to social expectations and therefore, we view them as bizarre.

P. Patience. Children with autism often have a great deal done for them or to them. If we are to convey to the child our belief in his capabilities, we must allow him the time to do things for himself. Our society tends to promote the expectation of a fast response. Children with autism may have a 15-20 second delay (or longer) in response time. That is a very long delay and requires lots of patience.

P. Perspectives. It is important to view behavior from a variety of perspectives (i.e. medical, sensory, communicative, etc.) and perhaps try various interventions. Any change in behavior (positive or negative) should first be viewed from a medical perspective. Some children display decreased hyperactivity and greater attentiveness during illness. Sometimes a behavior is an attempt to decrease pain. Sometimes we get caught in the trap of viewing all behavior from one perspective only. For example, my son was observed running his fingers along the brick wall in his classroom. Like many children with autism he has a history of sensory difficulties. This behavior was initially viewed as his need for sensory input. Further investigation revealed the true meaning of the brick wall. My son has a computer game that contains brick walls that can open to reveal hidden rooms. Once he was told there were no hidden rooms in the classroom, the "problem" was alleviated.

R. Rules. We all make sense of the world by developing rules to live by. The child with autism develops his own unique rules and lacks the communicative ability to tell you what those rules are. For example, a child with autism was sitting at a table having a snack. He suddenly jumped up from his chair and started screaming. Because the behavior was so sudden

216

and disconcerting, attention was focused on the child. A review of the environment revealed that the "snack" included crackers of a star shape. This child had developed a rule that crackers are round or square and this star shape broke his rule. It is a common occurrence for a child with autism to display unwanted behaviors in an attempt to convey that someone has broken a rule or that something is different.

E. Everything has to be taught and everything has to be specific working with a child with autism. In teaching my son to buy ice cream in a store, we broke it down into steps and daily repeated the routines. One day, we went into the store. David strode confidently to the counter and said "David wants vanilla." There was no clerk in sight – he was in the back of the store on the telephone. We had failed to teach David that the clerk needed to be present. What is obvious to most people is not to a child with autism. This includes communication. For example, I was taking some things out of the refrigerator. My son, David was nearby and I asked him to *"Close the door."* David left the room and closed the back door. Even though I was standing by an open refrigerator door, David did not understand. A child with autism does not attend to subtle environmental cues.

C. Choices. Making choices allows one to gain a sense of control over the environment. It is a step toward independence. Allow children with autism the opportunity to make choices whenever possible but be sure you are offering a choice. We sometimes use language to be polite that may be misinterpreted by a child with autism. "Would you like to go out to play now?" or *"Are you ready for lunch?"* implies a choice. Also remember that some children will respond with a *"yes"* to anything you say but not really want what you offer. Sometimes problems are created when choices are not allowed. One day, I received a call about a "problem behavior" for a young teenager with autism. It seems the teenager had taken to throwing his lunch in the trashcan rather than eating it. Further investigation revealed that the teacher was telling the teenager to eat his sandwich before he ate his dessert. This battle resulted in the lunch ending in the trashcan. A discussion with the mother revealed that the teenager normally ate his dessert before he ate his sandwich but always ate well and she wasn't concerned. Once the teacher understood this, he agreed that the teenager should be allowed the choice.

I. Inform. Tell a child with autism what is going to happen and when. This is particularly important when there is going to be a change in the schedule or the environment. The way the information is conveyed may vary depending on the child's needs. Sometimes pictures or lists are used. Some children can use clocks and calendars.

A. <u>Accommodations</u>. Although we all require accommodations for our needs, we often do not give the same respect to a child with a disability. When most children start preschool they take a favorite toy and enjoy a comforting hug from an adult. My son does not take his comfort in the same manner so he took a box and blanket to school. Although he started out in the box with a blanket over his head, he quickly adjusted and in the next few weeks the accommodation was removed. Accommodations may be a trampoline in the classroom and home, earphones while shopping or standing at the end of a line for a child sensitive to touch.

T. <u>Teach Social Rules and Expectations.</u> A child with autism has more than a language disability. He has a social disability. The child has to be taught not only how to socially interact but when. For example, we can teach a child to hug and kiss but we also need to teach when and with whom this is appropriate. Most children learn many things through observation but children with autism have to be taught specific social expectations. This may include using low voices in certain environments (i.e. library, movie theater) or refraining from socially inappropriate behaviors in public.

E. <u>Exercise</u>. A daily, vigorous exercise program is essential to any behavior program. There is increasing evidence that vigorous exercise is helpful to children with autism by reducing inappropriate behaviors and increasing their ability to concentrate.

Merritt, Cheryl S. December, 1993. <u>The Advocate</u>, Newsletter of the Autism Society of America, Inc. and Naiman, Daniel H. (editor) 1995 ***Autism: The Misunderstood Child***, <u>New Jersey Foster Parents Association.</u>

1994 DSM IV diagnostic criteria for Autistic Disorder, and Asperger's Syndrome from the Diagnostic and Statistical Manual of the American Psychiatric Association.

Autistic Disorder (299.00 DSM-IV)

The central features of Autistic Disorder are the presence of markedly abnormal or impaired development in social interaction and communication, and a markedly restricted repertoire of activity and interest. The manifestations of this disorder vary greatly depending on the developmental level and chronological age of the individual. Autistic Disorder is sometimes referred to as Early Infantile Autism, Childhood Autism, or Kanner's Autism.

A. A total of six (or more) items from (1), (2), and (3), with at least two from (1), and one each from (2) and (3):

1. Qualitative impairment in social interaction, as manifested by at least two of the following:
    *   Marked impairment in the use of multiple nonverbal behaviors such as eye to-eye gaze, facial expression, body postures, and gestures to regulate social interaction.
    *   Failure to develop peer relationships appropriate to developmental level
    *   A lack of spontaneous seeking to share enjoyment, interests, or achievements with other people (e.g., by a lack of showing, bringing, or pointing out objects of interest)
    *   Lack of social or emotional reciprocity
2. Qualitative impairments in communication as manifested by at least one of the following:
    *   Delay in, or total lack of, the development of spoken language (not accompanied by an attempt to compensate through alternative modes of communication such as gestures or mime)
    *   In individuals with adequate speech, marked impairment in the ability to initiate or sustain a conversation with others
    *   Stereotyped and repetitive use of language or idiosyncratic language
    *   Lack of varied, spontaneous make-believe play or social imitative play appropriate to developmental level

3. Restricted repetitive and stereotyped patterns of behavior, interests, and activities, as manifested by at least one of the following:
   - Encompassing preoccupation with one or more stereotyped patterns of interest that is abnormal either in intensity or focus
   - Apparently inflexible adherence to specific, nonfunctional routines or rituals
   - Stereotyped and repetitive motor mannerisms (e.g., hand or finger flapping or twisting, or complex whole-body movements)
   - Persistent preoccupation with parts of object

B. Delays or abnormal functioning in at least one of the following areas, with onset prior to age 3 years:

- Social interaction
- Language as used in social communication
- Symbolic or imaginative play

C. The disturbance is not better accounted for by Rett's Disorder or Childhood Disintegrative Disorder.

Asperger's Disorder (299.80 DSM-IV)

The essential features of Asperger's Disorder are severe and sustained impairment in social interaction and the development of restricted, repetitive patterns of behavior, interest, and activity. The disturbance must clinically show significant impairment in social, occupational, and other important areas of functioning. In contrast to Autistic Disorder, there are no clinically significant delays in language. In addition there are no clinically significant delays in cognitive development or in the development of age-appropriate self-help skills, adaptive behavior, and curiosity about the environment in childhood.

A. Qualitative impairment in social interaction, as manifested by at least two of the following:

- Marked impairment in the use of multiple nonverbal behaviors such as eye-to-eye gaze, facial expression, body postures, and gestures to regulate social interaction
- Failure to develop peer relationships appropriate to developmental level
- A lack of spontaneous seeking to share enjoyment, interests, or achievements with other people (e.g., by a lack of showing, bringing, or pointing out objects of interest to other people)
- Lack of social or emotional reciprocity

B. Restricted repetitive and stereotyped patterns of behavior, interests, and activities, as manifested by at least one of the following:

- Encompassing preoccupation with one or more stereotyped and restricted patterns of interest that is abnormal either in intensity or focus
- Apparently inflexible adherence to specific, non-functional routines or rituals
- Stereotyped and repetitive motor mannerisms (e.g., hand or finger flapping or twisting, or complex whole-body movements)
- Persistent preoccupation with parts of objects

C. The disturbance causes clinically significant impairment in social, occupational, or other important areas of functioning.

D. There is no clinically significant general delay in language (e.g., single words used by age 2 years, communicative phrases used by age 3 years)

E. There is no clinically significant delay in cognitive development or in the development of age-appropriate self-help skills, adaptive behavior (other than in social interaction), and curiosity about the environment in childhood.

F. Criteria are not met for another specific Pervasive Developmental Disorder or Schizophrenia.

2013 DSM-5 299.00 Autism Spectrum Disorder from the Diagnostic and Statistical Manual of the American Psychiatric Association

A. Persistent deficits in social communication and social interaction across multiple contexts
1. Deficits in social-emotional reciprocity, ranging, for example, from abnormal social approach and failure of normal back-and-forth conversation; to reduced sharing of interests, emotions, or affect; to failure to initiate or respond to social interactions.

2. Deficits in nonverbal communicative behaviors used for social interaction, ranging, for example, from poorly integrated verbal and nonverbal communication; to abnormalities in eye contact and body language or deficits in understanding and use of gestures; to a total lack of facial expressions and nonverbal communication.

3. Deficits in developing, maintaining, and understand relationships, ranging, for example, from difficulties adjusting behavior to suit various social contexts; to difficulties in sharing imaginative play or in making friends; to absence of interest in peers.

Severity is based on social communication impairments and restricted, repetitive patterns of behavior.

B. Restricted, repetitive patterns of behavior, interests, or activities, as manifested by at least two of the following, currently or by history

1. Stereotyped or repetitive motor movements, use of objects, or speech (e.g., simple motor stereotypes, lining up toys or flipping objects, echolalia, idiosyncratic phrases).

2. Insistence on sameness, inflexible adherence to routines, or ritualized patterns of verbal or nonverbal behavior (e.g., extreme distress at small changes, difficulties with transitions, rigid thinking patterns, greeting rituals, need to take same route or eat same food every day).

3. Highly restricted, fixated interests that are abnormal in intensity or focus (e.g., strong attachment to or preoccupation with unusual objects, excessively circumscribed or perseverative interests).

4.   Hyper- or hypo-reactivity to sensory input or unusual interest in sensory aspects of the environment (e.g. apparent indifference to pain/temperature, adverse response to specific sounds or textures, excessive smelling or touching of objects, visual fascination with lights or movement).

Severity is based on social communication impairments and restricted, repetitive patterns of behavior.
Symptoms must be present in the early developmental period (but may not become fully manifest until social demands exceed limited capacities, or may be masked by learned strategies in later life).
Symptoms cause clinically significant impairment in social, occupational, or other important areas of current functioning.
These disturbances are not better explained by intellectual disability (intellectual developmental disorder) or global developmental delay.
Intellectual disability and autism spectrum disorder frequently co-occur; to make comorbid diagnoses of autism spectrum disorder and intellectual disability, social communication should be below that expected for general developmental level.

References and Additional Reading

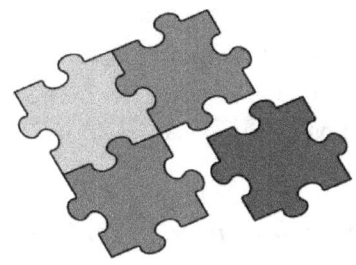

Anderson, Jeffrey, University of Utah. October 15, 2010. **"Diffusion Tensor MRI may yield autism diagnosis."** Retrieved from diagnosticimaging.com.

Baker, Candace (Director of Autism Interventions Center at Texas A&M International University). *Preparing Teachers for Students with Autism.* Retrieved on 2/9/2017 http://education.jhu.edu/PD/newhorizons/Journals/specialedjournal/BakerC.

Barnhill, G., Polloway, E. & Sumutka, B. (2011) *A Survey of personnel preparation practices in autism spectrum disorders.* Focus on Autism and Other Developmental Disabilities. Journals.sagepub.com.

Bauman, Margaret, M.D. (December 28, 1999). **New theories Help Explain Mysteries of Autism.** By Sandra Blakeslee. New York Times.

Chang, Heltz and Avila, Willian (Sept. 14, 2015). **"Special Needs Student Found Dead on School Bus. May have been Waiting for Instructions."** NBC4 News, Southern California.

Chen, JoAnne (April 3, 2011). **"Autism's Lost Generation,"** *Parade Magazine,* The News and Observer, Raleigh, N.C.

Courchesne, Eric, and Pierce, Karen. 2005. **"Why the frontal cortex in autism might be talking only to itself: local over-connectivity but long-distance disconnection."** Current Opinion in Neurobiology 15:225-230.

Curran LK, Newschaffer CJ, Lee LC, Crawford SO, Johnston MV, Zimmerman AW. Dec. 2007. *"Behaviors associated with fever in children with autism spectrum disorders.* Pediatrics 120(6):e1386-92.

Dager, S.R., L. Wang, S.D. Friedman, D.W. Shaw, J.N. Constantino, A.A. Artru, G. Dawson and J.G. Csernansky. *"Shape Mapping of the Hippocampus in Young Children with Autism Spectrum Disorder."* American Journal of Neuroradiology (AJNR) April 2007, 28(4) 672-677.

Dawson, Geraldine, University of Washington (2001 April 18). *"Mother is just another face in the crowd to autistic children."* Science Daily. Retrieved November 19, 2011, from http://www.sciencedaily.com.

Dawson, Geraldine and Rosanoff, Michael, MPH. 2/1/2011. **"Sports Exercise and the Benefits of Physical Activity for Individuals with Autism."** Autism Speaks. www.autismspeaks.org/sciencenews.

DeWeerdt, Sarah 13 May 2013. *"Long-term studies track how autism changes with age."* SFARI Simons Foundation Autism Research Initiative.

Frances, Allen, M.D. 2013. *Saving Normal: An insider's revolt against out-of-control psychiatric diagnosis, DSM-5, big pharma, and the medicalization of ordinary life.* New York: Harper Collins books.

Gazziniga, Michael S. 2015. *Tales from Both Sides of the Brain.* New York: Harper Collins.

Gazziniga, Michael S. 2011. *Who's in Charge? Free Will and the Science of the Brain.* New York: HarperCollins Publishers.

Gazziniga, Michael S. 1998. *The Mind's Past.* California: The Regents of the University of California.

Grandin, Temple and Panck, Richard. 2014. **The Autistic Brain: Helping Different Kinds of Minds Succeed.** New York, Houghton Mifflin Harcourt Publishing Company.

Grandin, Temple 2008. **The Way I See It: A Personal Look at Autism and Asperger's.** Texas: Future Horizons, Inc.

Grandin, Temple 1995. *Thinking in Pictures and Other Reports from my Life with Autism*. New York: Vintage/Random House.

Grandin, Temple and Catherine Johnson 2005. **Animals in Transition: Using the Mysteries of Autism to Decode Animal Behavior.** www.Harcourt Books.com.

Grandin, Temple and Catherine Johnson 2010. **Animals Make Us Human: Creating the Best Life for Animals.** New York: Houghton Mifflin Harcourt Publishing Company.

Greenberg, Gary 2014. *The Book of Woe.* New York: Penguin Group.

Haier, Richard J. 2014. **Increased Intelligence is a myth (so far).** Frontiers in Systems Neuroscience. 2014:8:34.

Hart, Charles 1989. *Without Reason: A Family copes with two generations of autism.* New York, Harper & Rowe Publications, Inc.

Iacoboni, Marco 2008, 2009. *Mirroring People*. New York: Picador.

Itard, Jean-Marc-Gaspart 1962 (originally published 1806). *The Wild Boy of Aveyron.* New York: Appleton-Century-Crofts.

Jacobson, Roni. August 27, 2015. *"Massive International Project Raises Questions about the Validity of Psychology Research."* Scientific American.

Kandel, Eric R. 2018. **The Disordered Mind: What Unusual Brains Tell Us about Ourselves**. New York: Farrar, Straus and Giroux.

Kanner, Leo 1943. *"Autistic Disturbances of Affective Contact."* (Nervous Child. 2:217-50). http://www.neurodiversity.com/library. Library of the History of Autism Research,, Behaviorism & Psychiatry.

Kanner, Leo 1971. *"Follow-up Study of Eleven Children Originally Reported in 1943."* (Journal of Autism & Childhood Schizophrenia 1971 Apr-June; 1(2): 119-45. http://www.neurodiversity.com/library.

Kennedy, Sara. 2014. *"Children in Nicaragua Teach Scientists About Language."* Hands and Voices. http://handsandvoices.org/articles.

Kline, Ami and colleagues. 2007. **"Social and Communication Abilities and Disabilities in Higher Functioning Individuals with Autism Spectrum Disorders: The Vineland and the ADOS."** Journal of Autism and Developmental Disorders 37:748-759.

LeDoux, Joseph. 2002. *Synaptic Self: How Our Brains Become Who We Are.* New York: Viking Penguin Group.

Levitt, Jennifer G., Hua Xua, and colleagues, University of California, Los Angeles, CA. October 20,2011. **"Autistic Brains develop more slowly than healthy brains, researchers say".** Science Daily. 11/17/2011 retrieved from www.sciencedaily.com.

Lord, Catherine and colleagues. March 2012. *A Multisite Study of the Clinical Diagnosis of Different Autism Spectrum Disorders.* Arch. General Psychiatry 69(3): 3060313.

Lovaas, O. Ivar 1987. *"Behavioral Treatment and Normal Educational and Intellectual Functioning in Young Autistic Children."* Journal of Consulting and Clinical Psychology 1987, Vol. 55, No. 1,3-9.

Lovaas, O. Ivar 1993. *"The Development of a Treatment Research Project for Developmentally Disabled and Autistic Children."* Journal of Applied Behavior Analysis 1993, 26, 617-630, Number 4 (Winter 1993).

Lord, C. and E. Schopler. 1989. *The Role of Age at Assessment, Developmental level and Time in the Stability of Intelligence Scores in Young Autistic Children.* Journal of Autism and Developmental Disorders. 19(4).

Medina, John. 2008. **Brain Rules: 12 Principles for Surviving and Thriving at Work, Home, and School.** Seattle, WA: Pear Press.

Mesibov, Gary B., Shea, Victoria, and Schopler, Eric. 2004. **The TEACCH Approach to Autism Spectrum Disorders.** New York: Springer Science&Business Media, Inc. permissions@wkap.com

Mesibov, Gary B. and Shea, Victoria .Nov. 24, 2009. *"The TEACCH Program in the Era of Evidence-Based Practice."* Springer.

Myers, Jennifer McIlwee, 2010. **How to Teach Life Skills to Kids with Autism or Asperger's**. Texas: Future Horizons. Email: info@FHautism.com; www.FHautism.com.

Nauert, Rick PhD (Senior News Editor) 11/8/2011. *"Diagnoses of Autism Spectrum Disorders lack Reliability"*. Psych Central News. http://psychcentral.com/news/2011/11/08.

National Research Council 2001. *Educating Children with Autism.* Committee on Educational Interventions for Children with Autism. Division of Behavioral and Social Sciences and Education. Washington, DC: National Academy Press.

Penney, Darby and Stastny, Peter 2008. *The Lives they Left Behind: Suitcases from a State Hospital Attic.* New York: Bellevue Literary Press.

Phillips, Michael M. 12/14/2013. *The Lobotomy Files/Family Scars: Torn by Choices Made a Lifetime Ago.* The Wall Street Journal.

Pierce, Karen; Haist, Frank; Sedghat, Farshad; Courchesne, Eric. (2004) **The brain response to personally familiar faces in autism: findings of fusiform activity and beyond.** Brain, 127 2703-2716.

Ramachandran, V.S. 2011. *The Tell-Tale Brain: A neuroscientists' quest for what makes us human.* New York: W.W. Norton & Company, Inc.

Ramachandran, V.S. 2004. *A Brief Tour of Human consciou5ness*. New York: Pearson Education, Inc.

Restak, Richard M. 1994. *The Modular Brain: How new discoveries in neuroscience are answering age-old questions about memory, free will, consciousness, and personal identity.* New York: Touchstone.

Ridley, Matt. 2015. **The Evolution of Everything: How New Ideas Emerge**. New York: HaarperCollins Publishers.

Roux Anne M., Shattuck, Paul T., Rast, Jessica E., Rava, Julianna A., Anderson, Kristy. *A National Autism Indicators Report: Transition into*

Young Adulthood. Philadelphia, PA. Life Course Outcomes Research Program. A.J. Drexel Autism Institute, Drexel University, 2015.

Schreibman, Laura; Geraldine Dawson, Aubyn C. Stahmr, Rebecca Landa, Sally J. Rogers, Gail G. McGee, Connie Kasari, Brooke Ingersoll, Ann P. Kaiser, Yvonne Bruinsma, Erin McNerney, Amy Wetherby and Alycia Halladay. 2015. *Naturalistic Developmental Behavioral Interventions: Empirically Validated Treatments for Autism Spectrum Disorder*. Journal of Autism and Developmental Disorders.

Seguin, Edward 2012 (originally published 1866*)*. **Idiocy and Its Treatment by the Physiological Method**. www.forgottenbooks.org.

Shorter, Edward 2000. *The Kennedy Family and the Story of MentalRetardation.* Philadelphia, PA: Temple University.

Silberman, Steve 2015. **Neurotribes: The Legacy of Autism and the Future of Neurodiversity.** New York: Avery an imprint of Penguin Random House LLC.

Spitz, Herman 1986. **The Raising of Intelligence: A Selected History of Attempts to Raise Retarded Intelligence.** New Jersey: Lawrence Erlbaum Associates.

Switzky, Harvey N. Greenspan, Stephen (editors). *What is Mental Retardation? Ideas for an Evolving Disability in the 21*[st] *Century*. American Association on Mental Retardation.

Trent, James W., Jr. 1994. *Inventing the Feeble Mind: A History of Mental Retardation in the United States.* University of California Press, The Regents of the University of California.

Trivedi, Bijal P. October 4, 2001. *"Scientists Identify a Language Gene."* National Geographic Today. http://news.nationalgeographic.com/news.

Valenstein, Elliot S. 2010. *Great and Desperate Cures: The Rise and Decline of Psychosurgery and Other Radical Treatments for Mental Illness*. University of Michigan.

Waldrop, Keri. (2017) **"Using Visual Structure for Medical Appointments."** TEACCH Carolina Living and Learning Center. Teach.com/CLLC/Carolina-living-and-learning-center.

Warren, Zachary, McPheeters, Melisssa L., Sathe, Mila, Foss-Feig, Jennifer H., Glasser, Allison, Veenstra-VanderWeele, Jeremy. March 2011. *"A systematic Review of Early Intensive Intervention for Autism Spectrum Disorders.* Pediatrics.

White, S. Williams and colleagues. 2007. "**Educational Placements and Service Use Patterns of Individuals with Autism Spectrum Disorders**". Journal of Autism and Developmental Disorders. 37:1410.

Yarnall, Polly A. M.Ed. *Current Interventions In Autism – A Brief Analysis.* Advocate, Autism Society of America: Nov-Dec. 2000.

Zikopoulos, Basilis, Ph.D., and Barbas, Helen, Ph.D., Boston University. (2010, November 11). Science Daily.

37th Report to Congress on the Implementation of the Individuals with Disabilities Education Act, 2015, U.S. Department of Education, Office of Special Education and Rehabilitative Services (OSERS), Washington, D.C.